PROBL
ana

PROBLEMS IN ANAESTHESIA
analysis and management

Stanley Feldman
BSc, MB, BS, FFARCS
*Consultant Anaesthetist, Westminster
Hospital, London*

William Harrop-Griffiths
MA, MB, BS, FFARCS
*Senior Registrar, Anaesthetics, St Mary's
Hospital, London*

Nicholas Hirsch
MB, BS, FFARCS
*Consultant Anaesthetist, The National
Hospitals for Nervous Diseases, London*

Heinemann Medical Books

Heinemann Medical Books
An imprint of Heinemann Professional Publishing Ltd
Halley Court, Jordan Hill, Oxford OX2 8EJ

OXFORD LONDON SINGAPORE NAIROBI IBADAN
KINGSTON

First published 1989

British Library Cataloguing in Publication Data

Feldman, Stanley
 Problems in anaesthesia
 1. Medicine. Anaesthesia
 I. Title   II. Harrop-Griffiths, William
 III. Hirsch, Nicholas
 617′.96

 ISBN 0–433–00424–X

Typeset by
Latimer Trend & Company Ltd, Plymouth
and printed by
M & A Thomson Litho Ltd,
East Kilbride, Glasgow

Contents

CONTENTS

Preface

The anaesthetist is presented with many problems during the course of anaesthesia and its subsequent recovery. Faced with the dilemma of how and when to respond to these events, the inexperienced anaesthetist may either be guided by protocols, and react in a mechanical, algorithmic fashion, or alternatively may evaluate the physiological significance of the changes and respond appropriately when he or she observes that the changes are likely to have serious consequences. The object of this book is to encourage the anaesthetist to adopt the latter approach and, instead of treating numbers such as pulse rate or blood pressure, to analyse changes in terms of the physiology of the patient's responses and the pharmacology of the drugs used. We aim to stimulate a rational approach to any corrective treatment rather than one based on preset criteria for active intervention inevitable in predetermined protocols. For this reason we have deliberately avoided giving specific criteria for active interference and corrective courses of action, leaving the anaesthetist free to make sensible adjustments. It is our belief that good anaesthetic practice necessitates selecting the best treatment for each individual patient based upon his or her pathological condition and physiological responses.

To this end we have analysed a variety of common anaesthetic problems in terms of their physiological or pathological significance. We have not attempted to give exhaustive lists to cover every possible cause and available treatment, but rather to direct the anaesthetist along constructive lines of enquiry and to outline sensible guidelines for treatment. This book is not therefore primarily concerned with the treatment of specific problems; its intention is rather to promote a method of thinking analytically about the cause, significance and effects of the physiological derangements identified as problems.

This book is aimed at various groups of anaesthetists. We hope to guide the student and the inexperienced anaesthetist

PREFACE

embarking on a career in the specialty towards a more thoughtful way of approaching problems that will inevitably be encountered during anaesthetic practice. We anticipate this book will assist those junior anaesthetists sitting the first part of the FFARCS examination and we hope the more experienced anaesthetist may find it useful as a basis for teaching this approach to anaesthetists in training.

Stanley Feldman,
William Harrop-Griffiths,
Nicholas Hirsch,
1989

Introduction

Don't panic!
There are certain generalizations that can be applied to the practice of anaesthesia which are both obvious and yet contain the accumulated experience of many years of practice. As with all generalizations there are exceptions, but these usually concern specific problems dictated by the patient's condition or the surgical needs.

1. The simpler the anaesthetic, the safer it will be. The more agents used, the more syringes on the trolley, the more complex the anaesthetic machine and the greater the number of infusions and catheters used, the more chance there is of a mistake occurring and the more difficult its correction becomes. Anaesthetic experience should start with the mastery of simple techniques using few anaesthetic agents, with each providing a specific effect.
2. Drugs should be used in doses that produce the desired effect; wherever possible they should be titrated against the patient's response to avoid a gross overdose. It is fundamentally bad pharmacological practice – although occasionally expedient anaesthetic usage – deliberately to administer an overdose of one drug to produce an effect which is, in pharmacological terms, a side-effect. For example, an overdose of an hypnotic drug will produce analgesia sufficient for some short procedures; an overdose of an analgesic drug may be used to produce hypnosis and high concentrations of volatile anaesthetic agents produce muscle relaxation.
3. The nearer patients are to the physiological norm, the safer they are. Removing patients' power of spontaneous respiration makes them more vulnerable. Artificial ventilation carries a small but definite mortality and it should

only be undertaken if indicated. Manipulation of other physiological variables out of their normal range, as occurs during induced hypotension, deliberate hypothermia, one-lung anaesthesia and extracorporeal circulation, all increase the hazard to the patient.

4. If a problem occurs, send for help early. The longer one leaves seeking more experienced assistance, the more difficult it becomes to diagnose and treat the problem. Nowhere is this better demonstrated than with intubation problems. The ideal situation is to recognize the potential problem before it occurs so that help and advice are available. Never attempt difficult manoeuvres single-handed; the presence of an untrained assistant is better than being totally isolated with a difficult problem to manage.

5. Don't panic! The first treatment for all problems is to ensure adequate oxygenation of the patient. There is seldom an immediate indication for drugs. Remember that there are relatively few options open to the anaesthetist – he or she can alter ventilation, change the gas mixture, give more fluids of one kind or another, increase or decrease the amount of central nervous depression, give muscle relaxants and on occasions give drug support to the circulation. Of these options it is the ventilatory control that is paramount. Nearly all avoidable anaesthetic catastrophes are primarily due to ventilation problems.

Cardiac arrest

Definition

The term 'cardiac arrest' implies a sudden failure of the heart to produce an effective output. Although cardiac arrest is usually due to ventricular fibrillation, asystole or electromechanical dissociation, without an ECG these three are indistinguishable. All produce a pulseless patient who requires cardiopulmonary resuscitation.

Physiological significance

The body cannot survive without perfusion of oxygenated blood and cardiac arrest is incompatible with life. It therefore constitutes the extreme medical emergency. Irreversible brain damage usually occurs when circulatory arrest lasts for more than a few minutes. However, a number of factors may influence the period available before cerebral damage occurs.

The degree of tissue oxygenation before cardiac arrest is important. If the patient was well perfused with fully saturated blood immediately prior to the arrest there may well be significant stores of oxygen in the blood, tissues, and in body water. This may allow a greater period of total circulatory arrest before irreversible tissue damage occurs.

Conversely, if the arrest was preceded by a period of poor oxygenation as a result of inadequate ventilation, ventilation with a gas mixture containing an inadequate oxygen concentration, or failing circulation, then the 'safe' period is reduced. Such problems are common before cardiac arrest in the anaesthetic context.

Hypothermia prolongs the period of safe hypoxia by decreasing tissue oxygen demand. It is said that for each degree centigrade fall in temperature, body metabolism falls by approximately 7 per cent.

CARDIAC ARREST

Once the circulation has been re-established the acid products of anaerobic metabolism will cause a metabolic acidosis. It is reasonable to correct this, at least in part. However, there are physiological risks associated with bicarbonate administration. Each 100 mmol of sodium bicarbonate infused will produce 2.24 litres of carbon dioxide. This crosses easily into cells and worsens intracellular acidosis. Bicarbonate (8.4 per cent) is also hyperosmolar and presents a significant sodium load.

Diagnosis

Pallor is often the first indication of cardiac arrest. Capillary refill is absent and the carotid pulse is lost. Breathing may continue for a short period but soon ceases. The ECG may show a wide variety of rhythms, but commonly ventricular fibrillation or asystole is present. Electromechanical dissociation may be associated with normal sinus rhythm. The diagnosis of cardiac arrest is therefore not primarily an ECG diagnosis. The blood pressure becomes unrecordable, and a capnograph shows zero end-tidal carbon dioxide. A pulse oximeter may reveal a rapid fall in oxygen saturation, followed by a failure to provide a reading.

Management

The patient should be placed on a hard surface. A precordial blow may reverse ventricular fibrillation or may initiate electrical activity in the case of asystole. It is essential to secure a clear airway, ventilate the lungs with oxygen, start external cardiac compression and establish a venous line. Defibrillation and drug therapy are all secondary to the early establishment of oxygenation and, using external cardiac compression, of a cardiac output. So long as this produces a carotid or femoral pulse there is time to consider specific treatments.

3

Details of cardiac resuscitation are found in most major textbooks of anaesthesia and medicine. Figure 1.1 contains the current recommendations of the Resuscitation Council of the United Kingdom.

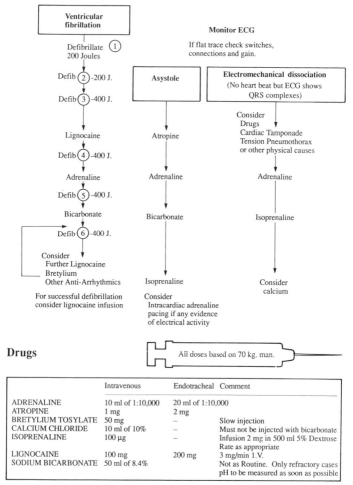

Fig. 1.1 The current recommendations for cardiopulmonary resuscitation (The Resuscitation Council UK)

	Intravenous	Endotracheal	Comment
ADRENALINE	10 ml of 1:10,000	20 ml of 1:10,000	
ATROPINE	1 mg	2 mg	
BRETYLIUM TOSYLATE	50 mg	–	Slow injection
CALCIUM CHLORIDE	10 ml of 10%	–	Must not be injected with bicarbonate
ISOPRENALINE	100 µg	–	Infusion 2 mg in 500 ml 5% Dextrose Rate as appropriate
LIGNOCAINE	100 mg	200 mg	3 mg/min I.V.
SODIUM BICARBONATE	50 ml of 8.4%		Not as Routine. Only refractory cases pH to be measured as soon as possible

Changes in pulse rate

BRADYCARDIA

Definition

Bradycardia can be defined as a pulse rate below 60 beats/min. However, in practical terms, it should be considered to be a heart rate that is sufficiently slow to cause concern for the adequate function of the patient's cardiovascular system, or a slowing of the rate indicating that adequate function may soon be compromised.

Few anaesthetists would disagree that a pulse rate below 40 beats/min requires treatment. However, there is a grey area between 40 and 60 beats/min where active intervention should be carefully considered in the light of the patient's cardiovascular status, coexisting drug therapy, age and the effect of the low pulse rate on other recordable variables.

Diagnosis

The diagnosis of bradycardia is commonly made by observation of the ECG, and the monitoring of a slow pulse rate. This differentiation is made as the pulse rate may occasionally be slower than the heart rate, particularly in situations where a proportion of heartbeats are abnormal, or where the heart rate is fast or irregular. In terms of circulatory adequacy, it is the pulse rate that is important.

Physiological significance

Except in the very fit individual, the stroke volume is unlikely to increase by more than 80–100 per cent of the resting value during exercise. There is therefore, in the normal patient, a degree of proportionality between the heart rate and the

5

cardiac output. In the young, the old, and in patients with valvular and myocardial disease, the stroke volume is more fixed, and so cardiac output tends to parallel closely the heart rate. Therefore, in all patients there comes a point during progressive bradycardia where increases in stroke volume become inadequate to maintain cardiac output at a level required to perfuse vital organs. The heart rate at which cardiac output becomes inadequate depends upon the cardio-vascular status of the individual, and in particular the patient's ability to increase stroke volume.

It is seldom that the anaesthetist is afforded the luxury of continuous cardiac output monitoring during an anaesthetic. It is therefore necessary to judge the adequacy of cardiac output by tissue perfusion, pulse pressure and the blood pressure. In most circumstances, provided tissue perfusion and blood pressure are maintained during bradycardia, there is no immediate cause for concern.

Bradycardia results in prolongation of the diastolic period. Patients with ischaemic heart disease may benefit from a modest fall in pulse rate as this allows more time for coronary perfusion, which occurs principally during diastole. This is especially true for hypertensive patients as subendocardial perfusion is limited to diastole. Patients with cardiac outflow obstruction, e.g. mitral and aortic valve stenosis, myocardial fibrosis and the cardiomyopathies, cannot easily increase their stroke volume. In this group of patients the cardiac output is proportional to the heart rate. As a result these individuals tolerate even moderate degrees of bradycardia badly. A similar state occurs in cardiac tamponade where ventricular filling is restricted.

The commonest form of bradycardia occurring during anaesthesia is sinus bradycardia (Fig. 1.2). In this situation the pulse rate is less than 60 beats/min and the ECG shows normal P waves, QRS complexes and T waves.

Bradycardias with abnormal ECG complexes may have more serious implications, indicating interference with con-

6

CHANGES IN PULSE RATE

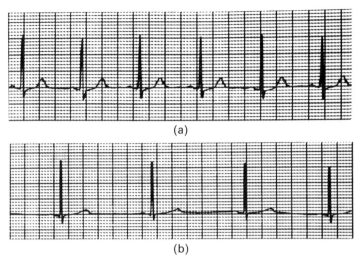

(a)

(b)

Fig. 1.2 (a) Sinus rhythm (b) Sinus bradycardia

duction within the heart (Fig. 1.3). Sinus arrest, nodal brady-cardia, second- and third-degree heart block or a slow idioven-tricular rhythm in the presence of atrial fibrillation or flutter may require treatment to avoid a profound, potentially refrac-tory bradycardia and a catastrophic fall in cardiac output.

Causes of bradycardia

Sinus or nodal bradycardia, usually attributed to vagal stimu-lation, is seen in the following situations:

A painful stimulus given to a lightly anaesthetized patient.
Surgical interventions to certain parts of the body:
external ocular muscles (the 'oculocardiac reflex')
carotid sinus
peritoneum and mesentery, especially stretching or
traction on the stomach and oesophagus
testicle and spermatic cord
anal stretch
cervical dilation

7

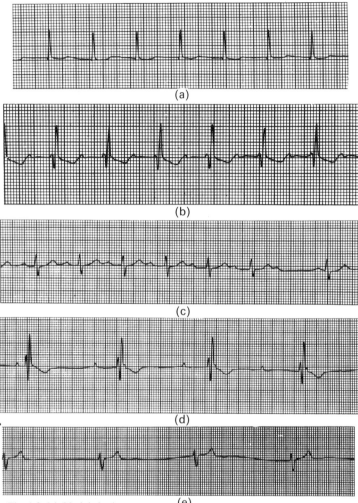

Fig. 1.3 (a) Nodal rhythm
(b) First degree atrioventricular block
(c) Second degree atrioventricular block (Wenkebach phenomenon, Morbitz type 1)
(d) Third degree atrioventricular block (complete heart block)
(e) Slow idioventricular rhythm

8

external auditory meatus

temporomandibular joint

A sudden increase in blood pressure can cause reflex brady-cardia, although this reflex is obtunded in deeper planes of anaesthesia.

A precipitate increase in intracranial pressure (Cushing's reflex).

Myocardial infarction or ischaemia involving the conducting tissues of the heart.

Hypothermia and the rapid intravenous infusion of cold fluid, usually through a central venous catheter, which may preferentially cool the sinoatrial node.

Hypoxia may initially produce sympathetic stimulation with an outpouring of catecholamines. However, due to its direct effect on the energy-sensitive conducting tissue of the heart, hypoxia will ultimately cause bradycardia. In neonates the heart rate invariably slows as a response to hypoxia – a similar effect is not uncommon in the elderly.

Drug effects are common causes of bradycardia:

Beta-blockers, digitalis glycosides, calcium antagonists.

Anticholinesterases in the absence of sufficient vagolytic treatment.

Deep anaesthesia with greater than two times the minimum aveolar concentration (MAC) with some volatile agents (especially halothane) is associated with bradycardia.

Opiates, most notably fentanyl and its cogeners, especially in combination with a muscle relaxant devoid of vagal blocking action, notably vecuronium and atracurium, have been associated with bradycardia and sinus arrest.

Suxamethonium, especially if a second dose is given within 4 min of the first.

Lignocaine, and other local anaesthetics.

Ecothiopate eyedrops.

Nodal bradycardia may be the result of hypoxia, hypercapnia, ischaemic heart disease or a combination of these. Heart block of any degree, is usually associated with ischaemic heart disease. Atrial flutter or fibrillation associated with a slow ventricular rate indicates a degree of heart block and may also be associated with overdose of digoxin or beta-blockers.

Management

Providing cardiac output is maintained at a level that ensures adequate tissue blood flow, bradycardia is unlikely to be life-threatening. However, it should alert the anaesthetist to the possibility of its progression to a point where the circulation will be compromised.

The adequacy of the patient's circulation may be assessed by a variety of observations, none of which is absolutely diagnostic on its own, but a combination may indicate a need for intervention. These include skin colour and warmth, pulse volume, blood pressure, pulse pressure, end-tidal carbon dioxide (at a constant minute ventilation), oxygen saturation as measured by a pulse oximeter, and mixed venous oxygen saturation.

Drugs should only be used if the circulation is considered to be inadequate, or if the bradycardia is worsening. First, consider if the bradycardia has an identifiable and reversible cause. The anaesthetist must ensure that the patient is adequately oxygenated. If the bradycardia has been the result of surgical stimulation, the anaesthesia may be too light and should be deepened. If in doubt as to the cause, the surgeons should be asked to suspend any procedure that may be producing vagal stimulation. If it is due to manipulation of the carotid sinus the reflex can be blocked by infiltration of the sinus nerve local anaesthetic.

If the bradycardia is drug-induced or has no identifiable and reversible cause, atropine 0.6–1.0 mg should be administered and repeated if necessary. Small doses of atropine, especially if given by intramuscular injection, may worsen the bradycardia due to central vagal stimulation.

If there is no response to atropine, 2.5–5 µg isoprenaline may be administered intravenously. Repeat this dose if necessary. If repeated doses are required to prevent serious bradycardia which is impeding adequate cardiac output, an isoprenaline infusion or cardiac pacing should be considered.

TACHYCARDIA

Definition

Tachycardia in an adult patient may be defined as a persistent pulse rate of over 100 beats/min. A more physiological description may consider tachycardia to be an increase in pulse rate in excess of that which is desirable for efficient myocardial and circulatory function.

Tachycardia may be diagnosed by palpation of an artery or observation of the ECG. In some situations, most notably atrial fibrillation, there may be a discrepancy between the heart rate seen on the ECG and the pulse rate as determined by palpation.

Physiological significance

Sedentary adults achieve the major part of their increase in cardiac output in response to exercise by increasing cardiac rate. The increased output parallels the increase in rate only as long as it is accompanied by a full stroke volume. As the rate increases, diastolic ventricular filling time falls, requiring increased atrial pressure to effect rapid ventricular filling. There comes a point at which this process fails, resulting in a fall in ventricular volume and diminished stroke volume. The increase in rate of contraction requires greater energy expenditure and this must be met by increased coronary perfusion.

However, an increase in cardiac rate is at the expense of diastole, during which much of the effective coronary perfusion occurs. Therefore tachycardia effectively decreases myocardial perfusion, especially to the vulnerable subendocardial vessels. As a result, the ratio of oxygen demand to oxygen availability increases and relative ischaemia occurs. This predisposes to dysrhythmias, and to a further fall in stroke volume, aggravating this potentially dangerous situation.

Causes of tachycardia

1. *Increased catecholamine secretion*
   Sympathetic stimulation secondary to hypoxia and hypercarbia.
   Central nervous system stimulation due to surgical stimulation under light or inadequate anaesthesia.
   Catecholamine-secreting tumours.
   Directly and indirectly acting sympathomimetic drugs.
2. *Decreased vagal tone*
   Drugs with vagolytic activity such as atropine, hyoscine, pancuronium, gallamine, etc.
3. *Reflex tachycardia*
   Compensatory in hypotensive states.
   High right atrial pressure (Bainbridge reflex) to compensate for low output of right ventricle or venous engorgement, e.g. overtransfusion.
   Myocardial ischaemia.
4. *Miscellaneous conditions*
   Hyperthermia, hyperthyroidism, mismatched blood transfusion, drug reactions, etc.
5. *Dysrhythmias*
   Atrial fibrillation and flutter, supraventricular tachycardias, ventricular tachycardias (Fig. 1.4).

CHANGES IN PULSE RATE

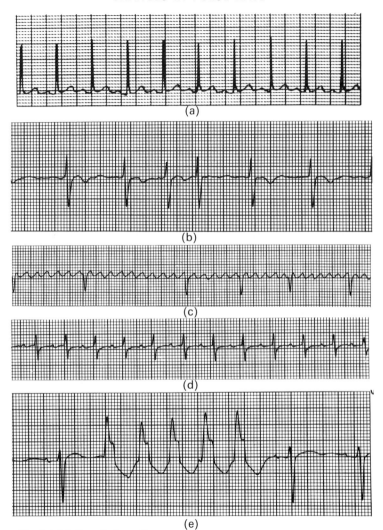

Fig. 1.4 (a) Sinus tachycardia
(b) Atrial fibrillation
(c) Atrial flutter
(d) Supraventricular tachycardia
(e) Ventricular tachycardia

13

Management

Before embarking on therapeutic intervention, the anaesthetist must assess whether the tachycardia has a pathophysiological basis, whether it requires treatment, whether it is likely to be amenable to treatment, and whether treatment of the tachycardia is likely to have a net benefit for the patient.

High pulse rates are physiological in neonates and small infants, and seldom lead to cardiac decompensation. In the elderly, tachycardia is physiological on exertion or stress as the ability to increase stroke volume is limited. However, unlike infants, elderly patients do not tolerate prolonged periods of tachycardia well, as the fall in myocardial oxygen availability is commonly exaggerated by coronary artery disease and the higher afterload imposed by a less compliant arterial system.

Tachycardia in a pyrexial patient can be an appropriate response to increased metabolic demands, and providing the tachycardia represents no threat to myocardial viability, management should be directed towards treating the cause of the pyrexia rather than the tachycardia itself. A lightly anaesthetized patient who develops a sinus tachycardia in response to a painful surgical stimulus may require further analgesia or a deepening of anaesthesia.

Which tachycardias should receive therapeutic intervention? There can be no hard and fast rules, but the following situations should provoke consideration of intervention:

1. When the tachycardia occurs in a patient with known ischaemic heart disease, assumed ischaemic heart disease as a result of age or its association with other medical conditions, or when the ECG suggests myocardial ischaemia.
2. Tachycardia associated with hypotension, which may indicate cardiac failure (provided it is not due to hypovolaemia), and tachycardia associated with hypertension in the presence of adequate anaesthesia.

3.   Tachydysrhythmias previously undiagnosed or occurring de novo during anaesthesia, or those diagnosed preoperatively which are increasing.

Providing the tachycardia is stable and is not interfering with cardiac function, and there is no evidence of myocardial ischaemia, there is no immediate need to intervene. Consideration should be given to the cause of the tachycardia, and if possible, steps should be taken to alleviate the cause. Specific drug treatment, though often useful, can occasionally worsen a situation and should not be embarked upon lightly. For instance, beta-adrenoceptor blockers are negatively inotropic, and when given to a patient who is tachycardic and hypotensive as a result of cardiac failure can have disastrous results. The development of a tachycardia can be seen as providing the anaesthetist with information about a physiological, pathological or pharmacological change that is occurring in the patient. It is the nature and treatment of this change which should be considered before taking therapeutic action to treat what is in effect a symptom of an underlying pathophysiological change.

Changes in blood pressure

Normal blood pressure is a continuously changing quantity and as such is difficult to define except in terms of function. However, a normal blood pressure may be considered to be one that produces an adequate perfusing pressure to meet the demands of the body without causing unnecessary demand upon the heart or damage to other organs. The average resting blood pressure of a young 70 kg adult is usually considered as 120/80 mmHg. A 30 per cent deviation would be considered outside the average normal range, although not necessarily pathological in that patient at that time.

Variations of greater than 30 per cent of the pre-induction pressure during the course of anaesthesia are common; they may be of a temporary nature and of little significance or they may herald impending catastrophic changes. In order to react appropriately, the anaesthetist must assess the likely cause and its significance before deciding what, if any, action is required.

HYPOTENSION

Physiological significance

Blood pressure is proportional to cardiac output and peripheral vascular resistance, and it is the variation in these latter two parameters that is responsible for changes in blood pressure. Compensatory mechanisms exist to maintain blood pressure within a relatively narrow range. However, significant changes in either cardiac output or peripheral vascular resistance will cause changes in blood pressure.

For normal function the tissues of the body require a supply of oxygen. The cardiovascular system serves this function by providing perfusion of vascular beds with oxygenated blood.

CHANGES IN BLOOD PRESSURE

The flow necessary to supply a tissue's requirements depends on the oxygen demand of that tissue. The flow through a vascular bed is proportional to the net perfusing pressure (the difference between the arterial and venous pressures) and is inversely proportional to the vascular resistance within that bed. Some organs of the body have the ability to autoregulate their flow, i.e. responding to changes in blood pressure by adjusting vascular resistance in order to maintain an adequate flow. However, there are limits to this capacity for autoregulation, and significant degrees of hypotension or hypertension will cause abnormally low or high blood flow respectively. Disease processes, for example arteriosclerosis, may affect the ability of a vascular bed to autoregulate effectively.

Hypotension caused by peripheral vasodilation will not necessarily cause a fall in tissue blood perfusion. Providing that cardiac output is maintained, and the blood pressure is not below the minimum necessary to perfuse organs, flow will be maintained.

There is no simple identifiable level of blood pressure that will be sufficient to perfuse the vital organs of all patients. The minimum safe blood pressure will vary greatly between patients, and even within the same patient will vary according to his or her current pathological and physiological status.

If tissue oxygen tensions could be measured it would be simple to determine whether oxygen demands were being met. However, as this is not practical, we have to depend on indirect indices such as skin colour, venous oxygen saturation and the outward signs of the normal function of each organ system.

Once tissue oxygenation becomes inadequate cell function becomes impaired. In the brain this is associated with impaired consciousness, as is sometimes seen during the hypotension produced by epidural anaesthesia, and irregular respiration – this can occur in patients during induced hypotension and is a valuable warning sign that the blood pressure is too low. In the heart this is associated with ECG changes, ischaemic changes affecting the ST segments and dysrhythmias. In the kidney

17

there is a reduction in urine formation (though this does not necessarily indicate tissue hypoxia; it may be due to lowered filtration pressure or water conservation).

Diagnosis

Hypotension is diagnosed after measuring the blood pressure by direct or indirect means. Certain patterns of hypotension may give a clue as to its cause, e.g. hypotension due to a fall in cardiac output (or more accurately, stroke volume) often results in a reduction in pulse pressure, i.e. the difference between systolic and diastolic pressures. Hypotension due solely to a fall in peripheral vascular resistance is characterized by a maintenance of pulse pressure.

The cause of the hypotension may be obvious. It may be deliberately induced or may follow the administration of a drug such as thiopentone which causes a transient fall in cardiac output or d-tubocurarine which frequently produces a fall in peripheral resistance. A brisk surgically induced haemorrhage followed by a fall in systolic pressure indicates the need for fluid replacement. A modest decrease in preload as a result of a head-up tilt of the operating table may be deliberately used to reduce bleeding.

It is when the hypotension is unrelated to either surgical or anaesthetic events that an attempt to elucidate its cause and its significance must be made. If invasive monitoring such as a Swan–Ganz catheter is being used, measurements of cardiac output and preload can be made, and peripheral vascular resistance can be calculated. However, when hypotension occurs under less well monitored conditions its cause can usually be deduced from simple observations and from available monitors.

Is hypotension due to a fall in peripheral resistance?

In this case the patient will be warm, vasodilated and usually pink (especially the veins at the back of the hand). The pulse pressure will be maintained at the expense of the diastolic value which will be low. Pulse volume as assessed by palpation will be adequate. Tachycardia is usually found; the pulse oxmeter will register normal oxygen saturation and the arteriovenous oxygen difference is seldom greatly increased.

Is the hypotension due to a fall in cardiac output?

The patient is likely to be vasoconstricted and may have central pallor. The pulse pressure will be narrowed with a reduction mainly in systolic value; pulse volume as assessed by palpation will be poor. The end-tidal carbon dioxide at constant minute ventilation will be reduced. A pulse oximeter usually shows a fall in saturation. The arteriovenous oxygen difference will increase, often causing a cyanotic tinge.

Aetiology

Fall in periperhal resistance

Common causes of a fall in peripheral vascular resistance include the following:

1. Almost all anaesthetic agents, particularly the volatile agents, result in a decreased peripheral vascular resistance which is proportional to their dosage. This may be due to a direct effect or to central vasomotor depression. The latter can also be caused by sedative agents and opiate analgesics. The difference between the blood concentration required for anaesthesia and that which will produce central autonomic depression is an index of its therapeutic ratio.
2. Histamine release stimulated by agents such as 2-tubocurarine and morphine, or subsequent to an anaphylactic or anaphylactoid reaction.

3. Drugs used for the treatment of hypertension, whether direct vasodilators, alpha-adrenoceptor antagonists, ganglion blockers or calcium channel blockers. Drugs given to induce hypotension during anaesthesia.
4. Autonomic blockade following subarachnoid, epidural or sympathetic block.
5. Hypercapnia and hyperthermia.
6. Local anaesthetic agents, both by a direct effect and following systemic absorption.

Fall in cardiac output

Causes of a fall in cardiac output due to a reduction in venous return include:

1. Intermittent positive pressure ventilation, particularly in conjunction with positive end-expiratory pressure.
2. Venodilation as part of generalized vasodilation for reasons listed above. This will have a pronounced effect on patients who were previously hypovolaemic due to haemorrhage, dehydration or other causes of low intravascular volume.
3. Operative blood or fluid loss.
4. Head-up tilt of the operating table.

Causes of a fall in cardiac output due to reduced cardiac function include:

1. Myocardial depression. Anaesthetic agents such as thiopentone and the inhalational agents, particularly halothane.
2. Other drugs include beta-adrenoceptor blockers, calcium channel blockers and local anaesthetics. Ischaemia, hypoxia, severe acidosis and alkalosis, and ionic imbalance cause myocardial depression, as may the withdrawal of inotropic agents if the patient has been receiving them for some time.

3. Dysrhythmias.
4. Pericardial tamponade.

Management

The cause of hypotension may be apparent from consideration of the anaesthetic and surgical situation and the use of clinical assessment and non-invasive monitoring. If a central venous or pulmonary artery catheter is being used, this may confirm the diagnosis. In general, hypotension due to vasodilation or reduced venous return will be associated with a falling central venous or pulmonary capillary wedge pressure. Hypotension due to poor cardiac function may be associated with a rising central venous pressure or pulmonary capillary wedge pressure.

If such invasive monitoring is not being used, the response of the blood pressure to the infusion of 500 ml of fluid may give useful information. Hypotension due to reduced venous return or vasodilation will respond to this, though perhaps only briefly, whereas hypotension due to poor cardiac function is unlikely to respond to this manoeuvre. Tipping the patient head-down may yield the same responses, and does not put patients with poor cardiac function at the risk of volume overload.

If the hypotension is not severe, and the cause is known to be self-limiting and likely to be of short duration, it may not be necessary to take any action other than to continue monitoring the patient carefully.

If it is felt that therapeutic action is required, simple expedients such as ensuring adequate ventilation, increasing the inspired fraction of oxygen, tipping the table head-down and reducing the inspired concentration of inhalational agents may suffice. However, if an identifiable and reversible cause for significant hypotension is found, the appropiate action should be taken.

Vasoconstrictors such as ephedrine, methoxamine and

21

metaraminol should only be used when vasodilation is known to be the cause of the hypotension, and further intravenous volume has been given, or is felt to be undesirable. The use of vasoconstrictors to treat hypotension due to poor cardiac function is not recommended.

In the case of poor cardiac function as a result of myocardial depression due to a cause that is not easily remediable, inotropes may be necessary. The choice of inotrope will depend on the situation and personal preference. Dopamine remains a popular agent, and at the lower end of the dosage scale maintains or improves renal perfusion.

HYPERTENSION

Physiological significance

Hypertension during anaesthesia is usually the result of increased peripheral vascular resistance. Rarely, it may be due to increased cardiac output, often associated with an increase in venous return.

If the hypertension is the result of peripheral vasoconstriction it will reduce tissue perfusion, resulting in hypoxia and acidosis. The autoregulation of the cerebral circulation protects the brain against modest increases in perfusion pressure but this may fail or be overwhelmed at very high pressures. Protective rises in cerebrovascular resistance may cause cerebral ischaemia, whilst excessive pressure may cause cerebral haemorrhage.

Left ventricular work and concomitant myocardial oxygen demand increase to overcome the increased afterload of hypertension. Unless there is an increase in diastolic coronary perfusion time, the high intraventricular pressures generated during systole will cause a reduction in subendocardial oxygenation. It is essential that the increased work of the ventricle should be met by increased subendocardial perfusion, hence the danger of a simultaneous increase in blood pressure and cardiac rate. In the presence of established coronary artery disease the ability to increase perfusion to meet the increased oxygen demand associated with hypertension is limited and as a result ischaemia, dysrhythmias and infarction may occur.

Aetiology

Causes of acute increases in peripheral vascular resistance include the following:

1. Catecholamine secretion: anaesthesia that is too light causing a significant sympathetic response, hypoxia, hypercarbia, surgical stimulation of adrenal glands or other functioning sympathetic tissue, instability of autonomic nervous system, denervation hypersensitivity, phaeochromocytoma.
2. Drug effects: catecholamines, sympathomimetic agents, vasopressin, Syntocinon. In addition certain drugs such as cocaine and pancuronium inhibit the uptake of endogenously secreted adrenalin, causing an exaggerated hypertensive response to painful stimuli in light anaesthesia.
3. Renal effects: Conn's syndrome, renin secretion following acute renal ischaemia.
4. Miscellaneous: mismatched blood transfusion (possibly renally mediated), toxaemia of pregnancy.

The responses to the above of previously hypertensive patients may be exaggerated.

Management

By far the commonest cause of hypertensive episodes during anaesthesia is as a response to painful stimulation or laryngoscopy indicating too light a plane of anaesthesia. In the absence of any other pre-existing pathology which may predispose to an overactive autonomic state, a rise in systolic and diastolic blood pressure, usually associated with a rise in cardiac rate, in response to surgical stimulation suggests the need for more effective analgesia or deeper anaesthesia.

The hypertension associated with hypoxia and hypercarbia is mediated by catecholamine release. Tachycardia is a prominent sign but, especially if the hypoxaemia is severe, it will soon give way to bradycardia and dysrhythmias. Hypercarbic hypertension is often associated with a flushed sweaty skin in lighter planes of anaesthesia.

If anaesthesia and analgesia are felt to be adequate, and no other remediable cause of hypertension is present, and if the systolic pressure rises to life-threatening levels, the cautious use of antihypertensive agents may be employed. We recommend that the novice anaesthetist should not use these agents without careful consideration of other causes and consultation with, or supervision by, an experienced anaesthetist as they all carry serious side effects and have potentially serious physiological consequences.

Severe episodic hypertension, whether or not it is associated with tachycardia, and especially if it follows pressure in the renal area, suggests phaeochromocytoma. Although this tumour is not common (occurring in about 0.5% of hypertensive patients), failure to recognize it as a cause of the hypertension may be fatal. Untreated phaeochromocytomas carry a high perioperative mortality. Diagnosis depends upon demonstrating vanillylmandelic acid in the blood and urine, a test not suited to conditions of acute surgery. If this condition is suspected, the surgery should be postponed if at all possible. In emergency surgery alpha- and beta-adrenoceptor blocking agents combined with electrolyte infusion to expand the plasma volume are useful to control rises in blood pressure and heart rate. Direct intra-arterial blood pressure monitoring is essential in this condition if rapid changes in arterial pressure are not to be missed.

Dysrhythmias

Definition

Dysrhythmia may be defined as a cardiac rhythm that differs from normal sinus rhythm. The incidence of dysrhythmias during anaesthesia varies from 16 per cent in patients with no history of ischaemic heart disease to 34 per cent in patients with known heart disease. The high incidence of abnormal cardiac rhythm makes ECG monitoring during anaesthesia mandatory.

Physiological significance

The significance of dysrhythmias in anaesthetic management has two facets. Firstly, a change of rhythm often indicates a change in the patient's physiological status, alerting the anaesthetist to a possible further deterioration. Secondly, the dysrhythmia itself may have adverse effects on cardiac function and myocardial status.

A variety of physiological changes can affect cardiac rhythm. Airway obstruction or deep anaesthesia in the spontaneously breathing patient can cause hypoventilation and thus hypercapnia, which in turn causes abnormal cardiac rhythms. Hypoxaemia and significant acidosis or alkalosis, hypokalaemia and hyperkalaemia, hypothermia and hyperthermia can all be reasons for a change in cardiac rhythm. Dysrhythmias may be associated with light anaesthesia, the onset or worsening of myocardial ischaemia, or may be due to the effect of drug therapy, or of the combination of drugs, e.g. adrenalin and halothane or surgical stimulation to sensitive areas or direct manipulation of the heart. Such physiological and pharmacological influences are common during anaesthesia, and the change in cardiac rhythm should initiate the search to identify such a cause.

Most dysrhythmias will cause a decrease in cardiac output and blood pressure and a decrease in myocardial efficiency, necessitating an increase in myocardial oxygen utilization for a given stroke volume. A patient who has previously been in sinus rhythm and then develops a nodal rhythm may suffer a fall in cardiac output due to the loss of the atrial contribution to ventricular filling, although frequently it will be without significant clinical effect. If the heart rate exceeds 160 beats/min, even in the previously healthy adult patient, the greatly shortened diastole will allow less time for ventricular filling and cardiac output will fall. A tachydysrhythmia also allows less time for diastolic coronary perfusion, and yet increases the myocardial oxygen demand so that patients with coronary artery disease may rapidly develop myocardial ischaemia. Ventricular fibrillation, asystole, and often ventricular tachycardia may result, causing insufficient cardiac output to sustain life, and the development of these dysrhythmias constitutes cardiac arrest (see p. 2).

Diagnosis

The diagnosis of a dysrhythmia can often be suggested or made by the simple palpation of the pulse. However, confirmation must be sought from an ECG. Lead II is recommended for the detection of dysrhythmias as it most reliably provides adequate amplitude and morphology of both P waves and QRS complexes.

Management

If the dysrhythmia is immediately life-threatening (i.e. is not associated with a palpable pulse), the anaesthetist's priority lies with establishing a clear airway, giving 100 per cent oxygen and establishing a circulation, with external cardiac massage.

The anaesthetist should seek a physiological or pharmacological cause for the change in cardiac rhythm; correction of this

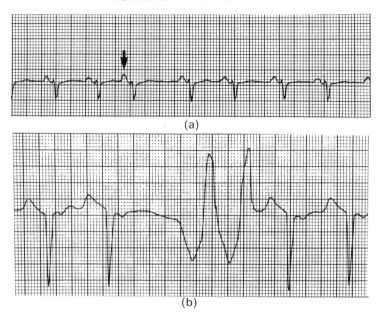

Fig. 1.5 (a) Atrial ectopic beat
        (b) Ventricular ectopic beats

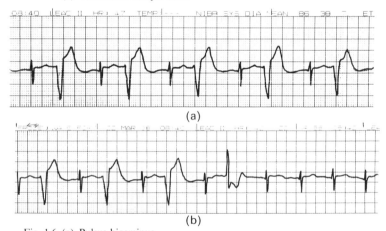

Fig. 1.6 (a) Pulsus bigeminus
        (b) Effect of hyperventilation in correcting pulsus bigeminus

will usually cause the dysrhythmia to revert. The commonest dysrhythmias are atrial and ventricular ectopic beats, nodal rhythm and pulsus bigeminus (Figs. 1.5 and 1.6). They are rarely the cause of significant cardiovascular decompensation and seldom justify pharmacological correction. Only after the anaesthetist is satisfied that the patient is not hypoxic, hypercapnic or too lightly anaesthetized and that the frequency or severity of the dysrhythmias is seriously affecting cardiac function or may lead to more serious dysrhythmias, should pharmacological action be considered.

Ventricular ectopic beats will usually respond to intravenous lignocaine or beta-blocker administration. Nodal rhythm may revert to sinus rhythm after intravenous atropine and bigemini often respond to lowering the $P_a\text{CO}_2$ by hyperventilation (Fig. 1.6). The rate of atrial fibrillation should slow in response to cardiac glycosides, and supraventricular tachycardia, if unresponsive to eyeball and carotid body massage, may revert after verapamil. DC cardioversion to correct supraventricular tachycardia, ventricular tachycardia or atrial fibrillation may be used after careful consideration.

Haemorrhage

Definition

There are various rules of thumb to indicate when surgical blood loss has reached sufficient magnitude to require replacement of volume. Traditionally, a patient who suffers an acute loss of 20 per cent of circulating volume is said to require blood transfusion. In practice much depends on the patient's preoperative haemoglobin, fluid balance, age, myocardial status, and the likelihood of continued blood loss after surgery is complete. It must be emphasized that the decision to transfuse blood should not be made lightly, but as a result of careful evaluation of the benefits to the patient at that particular time.

Physiological significance

As haemoglobin is the principle means for the distribution of oxygen from the lungs to the tissues it follows that the concentration should be such that it will meet that demand without excessive strain on the heart.

Provided adequate oxygenation takes place, the haemoglobin concentration has to fall to below 10 g/dl before cardiac output needs to increase significantly to supply the oxygen demands of the tissues. Indeed, haemodilution reduces afterload and hence decreases cardiac work. This situation is less satisfactory postoperatively when oxygen demand increases above basal levels and oxygenation may be impaired. The use of large amounts of stored blood may also be counterproductive, as even though the haemoglobin concentration will be increased, stored blood gives up oxygen less readily to the tissues, due to a shift to the left of the oxyhaemoglobin dissociation curve caused by lower 2.3 DPG (Fig. 1.7). This, coupled with the inevitable fluid load given, may impose a burden on the circulation. Blood transfusion also carries

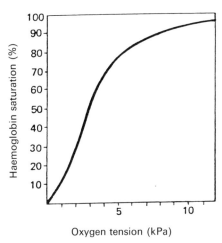

Fig. 1.7 The oxyhaemoglobin dissociation curve. The curve is shifted to the left by a variety of factors which include increased pH, decreased temperature and a lowered intracellular concentration of 2.3 DPG

certain other risks to the recipient of infection, reactions, mismatched transfusions and possible depression of the immune response.

Diagnosis and management

That surgical blood loss is occurring is usually self-evident. However, it is easy to underestimate its magnitude.

Swab weighing is useful provided that swabs are weighed soon after being discarded by the surgeon, and the necessary weighing and calculations are performed accurately. Measurement of the volume of blood in the sucker bottle is also helpful. If large volumes of irrigation fluid are used, the retrieval of this fluid should be included in calculations. Overall, underestimation of blood loss is likely with these methods due to failure to account for blood on the surgeon's gown, drapes and floor. It is notoriously difficult to estimate the amount of blood lost during transurethral prostatectomy due to dilution in the irrigation fluid.

31

Measurement of central venous pressure can be very useful to assess the effect of volume loss from the circulation, and to judge the adequacy of replacement. However, intravascular volume is not the only determinant of central venous pressure and care must be exercised in its interpretation (see p. 43). The complications associated with the insertion and use of central venous catheters are such that they should only be used when volume losses are likely to be large or rapid, or where there exist other indications for their use.

Loss of volume from the circulation during surgery is not just due to haemorrhage. Large volumes of fluid can be lost as plasma, into the third space, as water vapour by exhalation, or by evaporation.

The anaesthetist should assess the extent of blood loss during a surgical procedure from observation of the operative site and measurements of loss from swab and sucker calculations, while estimating the degree of loss of fluid not containing blood cells. It is important not to await the signs of hypovolaemia in the patient before initiating blood transfusion, although even in experienced hands it is not always possible to avoid this. The aim should be to keep pace with volume loss from the circulation. It is common practice to initiate fluid therapy with crystalloid or colloid, giving blood when the anaesthetist deems appropriate.

Some anaesthetists find it useful to allow the patient's haemoglobin concentration or haematocrit to approach a target value. Haematocrit estimations are a useful aid to this approach, though even without them, the presumption that the loss of 1 unit of blood from a 70 kg patient will, if the volume is replaced with fluid not containing red blood cells, reduce haemoglobin concentration by approximately 1 g/dl, and vice versa, may be used. This target value may be set after consideration of the patient's age, preoperative haemoglobin concentration, concurrent diseases and likelihood of continuing postoperative blood loss.

While considering blood transfusion during an operation,

the anaesthetist should be mindful of its dangers. These include:

1. Overtransfusion: this is most likely to cause problems in patients with poor myocardial reserve, those with non-compliant vascular systems (arteriopaths and the elderly), and young infants for whom a small amount of blood may represent a large proportion of the normal circulating volume.
2. Transfusion reactions: these can vary from mild pyrexia and rashes to haemolytic responses, coagulopathy and renal failure and cardiovascular collapse. The more serious reactions are often heralded by changes in blood pressure and pulse rate. Management includes stopping blood transfusion and responding to cardiovascular problems. Renal function can be impaired due to intravascular coagulation, hypotension and free haemoglobin in the renal tubules. For this reason, monitoring of urine output is important, and some authorities recommend the use of diuretics to increase renal blood flow and diuresis.
3. Hypothermia: a modest fall (to 34°C) in core temperature is seldom harmful in anaesthesia, although on rewarming shivering will greatly increase oxygen demand. Rapid transfusion with cold blood may produce sinus bradycardia and depress cardiac output due to its early contact with the right ventricle and the sinoatrial node. Blood warmers are useful if large volumes of fluid are transfused, and are also important when transfusing neonates and elderly patients whose response to hypothermia is impaired in comparison with a healthy young adult.

Blood is an expensive and potentially dangerous fluid. Its administration should always be the result of a full consideration of the advantages and the possible dangers that may result from its use.

Anaemia

Definition

Anaemia may be defined as a lowering of the haemoglobin concentration in the blood to below the normal range for the age and sex of the patient. It can be due to a reduction in the red blood cell count due to failure of haemopoiesis, excessive rate of destruction of red blood cells, or blood loss followed by physiological or iatrogenic replacement with fluid deficient in red blood cells.

Physiological significance

The tissues of the body require oxygen to supply their metabolic needs. The term 'oxygen flux' describes the total amount of oxygen available to the tissues per unit of time (Fig. 1.8). If the oxygen-carrying capacity of the blood is reduced by a fall in haemoglobin concentration, then in order to maintain the oxygen flux the patient must increase cardiac output or oxygen extraction. If it is not possible to compensate fully due to the extent of the anaemia or due to cardiac dysfunction, oxygen flux will decrease and tissue hypoxia may result. The extent to which an individual can compensate for anaemia is therefore dependent to a large extent on his or her cardiovascular status

---

$$\text{OXYGEN FLUX (in ml/min)} = \frac{Q \times SaO_2 \times Hb \times 1.39}{10}$$

Where: Q = Cardiac output in litres/min
SaO_2 = Arterial oxygen saturation in per cent
Hb = Haemoglobin concentration in mg/dl
1.39 = Oxygen capacity of haemoglobin in ml/g

Fig. 1.8 The simplified oxygen flux equation

and oxygen requirements. Under general anaesthesia, especially associated with artificial ventilation, the basal oxygen requirement of the body may be reduced by 30–35 per cent.

Haemodilution anaemia decreases the viscosity of blood and thereby increases flow through a vascular bed at the same perfusing pressure. This allows the heart to maintain the same cardiac output with less work. This decrease in the workload of the ventricles may increase the ability of the heart to meet increased cardiac output without raising its oxygen demand disproportionately. However, below a haematocrit of around 30 per cent, and in conditions other than complete rest, this benefit is outweighed by the increased cardiac output required to meet the body's oxygen demand.

Diagnosis and treatment

The diagnosis of anaemia is made from estimation of the haemoglobin content of the blood, but the interpretation of the result and the best method of correcting the anaemia requires consideration of the physiological effect it is having upon the patient. The possibility of an increased oxygen demand or blood loss occurring as a result of anaesthesia and surgery must be weighed against the benefits and disadvantages of preoperative blood transfusion to correct the condition.

The benefit of blood transfusion for the anaemic patient lies in the increased oxygen-carrying capacity of the blood. However, in the fit, well compensated individual with a moderate degree of anaemia who is scheduled for minor surgery, this benefit may not outweigh the risks of blood transfusion. These risks include transfusion reactions, infection, volume overload, hyperkalaemia and hypothermia. In contrast, the significantly anaemic patient, showing symptoms and signs of cardiac ischaemia and decompensation, who is scheduled for a procedure which will entail significant blood loss, will almost certainly benefit from careful blood transfusion in the days preceding surgery. Between these two extremes are patients for whom the risks and benefits must be considered, and a management decision taken on this basis.

There are no universal criteria for blood transfusion, though traditionally a haemoglobin of 10 g/dl is the watershed for postponement of a case pending restitution of a normal haemoglobin. This should not be taken as an absolute rule. For instance, patients with chronic renal failure commonly have a haemoglobin of considerably less than this value; most are well compensated for this level of anaemia, are unlikely to maintain a higher haemoglobin for any significant length of time, and are at considerable risk from the volume and potassium load that transfusion with stored blood could involve (Fig. 1.9). The 'rule of 10' should therefore not be seen as a incontrovertible physiological and medicolegal dictate, but simply as a level below which the anaesthetist should give particular consideration to the question of preoperative therapy aimed at treating the anaemia.

If preoperative transfusion is considered necessary, its timing is important. The reduced levels of 2,3-diphosphoglycerate in stored blood cause a shift to the left in the haemoglobin dissociation curve, thereby reducing oxygen availability to the tissues. It takes time for the body to correct this biochemical lesion and therefore it is commonly recommended that transfusion should take place at least 48 hours prior to surgery.

If time permits, management of anaemia should include discovering its cause. Transfusion should not be regarded as the panacea for low haemoglobin levels. Iron deficiency is the commonest cause of anaemia, and patients with iron deficiency anaemia presenting for non-urgent surgery should receive iron therapy rather than transfusion.

Caution should be exercised during preoperative transfusion in those patients who tolerate a large volume load poorly. The transfusion of packed red blood cells or plasma-reduced blood in conjunction with the administration of diuretics will decrease the degree of volume load.

A bag of blood contains

Approximately 450 ml whole blood + 63 ml citrate phosphate dextrose solution at 2–6 degrees centigrade.

pH   = 6.9
pCO_2 = 140 mmHg
HCO_3 = 11 mmol/l

plasma potassium =   21 mmol/l
plasma lactate   =   179 mmol/l
active platelets: none
factors V and VII: less than 20%

Fig. 1.9 The contents of a bag of blood after three weeks storage

Finally, it should be noted that it is too easy to assume that the patient's anaemia is due to the pathology for which surgery is required. It should always be borne in mind that the anaemia may be due to haemolysis, a haemoglobinopathy, depression of erythropoiesis or bleeding from a coincident pathology which may complicate anaesthesia and recovery.

Embolism

Definition

Embolism implies the blockage of a blood vessel by material that has been carried to that place in the bloodstream. For the anaesthetist, pulmonary embolism is the most important type of embolism; only this will be considered here.

Physiological significance

Because of the particular importance of the pulmonary artery in the oxygenation of blood in the lungs, pulmonary embolism has very serious consequences. It is probable that small emboli are frequently filtered in the pulmonary capillary bed but due to the ease with which parallel vessels can open up in the vascular bed in the lungs, these have little physiological significance. However, recurrent emboli may lead to pulmonary hypertension.

Once the main pulmonary artery or, more commonly, the right or left pulmonary arteries are even partially blocked there is enormous back pressure on the thin-walled right ventricle. Acute cor pulmonale usually occurs when 50 per cent of the pulmonary vasculature is obstructed. The failure of blood to reach beyond the embolus leads to acute ventilation/perfusion mismatch which, should the patient survive, may result in inadequate oxygenation. The reduction in venous return to the left side of the heart causes a reduction in the cardiac output, which in turn reduces coronary filling at a time when right ventricular work is increased.

Classic causes of pulmonary embolus during surgery are detachment of clots in the legs or pelvic veins following immobilization, amniotic fluid emboli in obstetric patients, fat emboli after trauma or during surgery to the long bones, and air embolus (see below).

Diagnosis

Pulmonary embolism occurring during anaesthesia is characterized by dysrhythmias, tachycardia and increasing cyanosis despite ventilation of the lungs with oxygen-rich mixtures of gases. Bronchospasm may rarely occur. Often, if the pulmonary embolism is large, the resulting shunt means that even ventilation with 100 per cent oxygen produces no improvement in oxygenation. If the patient is breathing spontaneously, he or she may demonstrate 'air hunger'. The patient will show the signs of falling cardiac output, the end-tidal carbon dioxide will drop, as will oxygen saturation, and the ECG may show the hallmarks of right heart strain.

Management

Management of pulmonary embolism includes maintenance of adequate oxygenation, if possible, by increases in inspired oxygen concentration and appropriate treatment of cardiovascular disturbances. If deep venous thrombosis is thought to be an aetiological factor, anticoagulation and streptokinase administration should be considered.

Air Embolism

Air entering the venous system will collect in the heart and, if it is large in volume, it will prevent effective right ventricular contraction. Air may enter the circulation during operations involving the veins in the head, neck and thorax in patients in a head-up position, and the pelvis, especially if the patient is in the Trendelenburg position. It may occur following gas insufflation during laparoscopy and during neurosurgical procedures, especially those performed in the sitting position. Air embolism is a risk during the insertion and use of any intravascular catheter, but particularly with central venous and pulmonary artery catheters. It is more likely in patients breathing spontaneously than in those being ventilated artificially, due to the lower venous pressure.

Physiological significance

The adult ventricular capacity is about 60 ml. If this was suddenly and totally replaced with air it would completely prevent effective ejection of blood, resulting in a frothy mixture which would be inefficiently expelled into the pulmonary artery. It is doubtful if less than 10 ml of air would cause more than a transient fall in stroke volume, especially if it enters slowly through a peripheral vein.

However, if a septal defect is present in the heart (this is most commonly a patent foramen ovale), even a small amount of air entering the left ventricle may travel to the brain with serious consequences – paradoxical embolus.

Diagnosis and management

Awareness of the possibility of air embolism and a catastrophic fall in cardiac output will suggest the diagnosis. Auscultation over the precordium may reveal the classical millwheel murmur. In neurosurgery, a precordial Doppler probe is often used, and if air passes through the heart, a rushing noise is heard. End-tidal carbon dioxide will fall, and the patient may develop hypotension and dysrhythmias.

If air embolism occurs, further entry of air through the probable route should be prevented, the patient should be placed in the left lateral, head-down position and ventilated with 100 per cent oxygen. If a right atrial catheter has been placed, air may be aspirated through this. If the clinical picture of cardiac arrest occurs, cardiopulmonary resuscitation should be initiated. In extreme emergency and with certain diagnosis it has been recommended that a large-bore needle should be placed percutaneously into the right ventricle and vigorously aspirated.

Changes in central venous pressure

Diagnosis

Before making a firm diagnosis of a rise or fall in central venous pressure (CVP), care must be taken to ensure that the change observed is not derived from technical sources of variation or error, of which some common examples are listed below:

1. The readings should be taken from a patent catheter lying within one of the great veins in the thorax or the right atrium. Absolute confirmation of this can only be acquired by radiographic or electrocardiographic means, or by direct visualization during surgery. However, correct placement is commonly achieved with techniques using the subclavian or internal jugular veins, while it is less common via the external jugular, femoral, basilic or cephalic veins. Measurements from catheters in extrathoracic veins cannot be relied upon in absolute terms, though they may on occasion give useful information concerning trends in the CVP.

2. The waveform of the observed CVP should be compatible with correct catheter placement, i.e. it should show variations with both cardiac and respiratory cycle (Fig. 1.10). The meniscus in a water manometer column should move freely, and the trace on an oscilloscope or similar monitor should be dynamic. Even though the catheter is correctly placed, damping of the CVP, and hence potential erroneous results, may ensue if the end of the catheter is against a vein wall or if it is kinked. Large swings of the meniscus and pressures over 25 cm H_2O suggest that the catheter is in the right ventricle.

3. Changes in the point of reference chosen for the CVP (i.e.

41

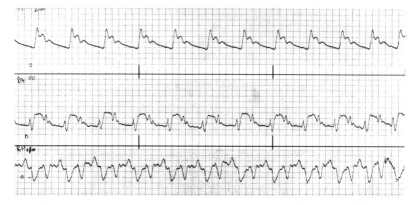

Fig. 1.10 Venous pressure monitoring: upper trace, arterial pressure; middle trace, pulmonary artery pressure; lower trace, central venous (right atrium) pressure showing negative phase during inspiration

the point to which the monitoring apparatus is 'zeroed') will produce spurious changes in the CVP. It is therefore important to be consistent in the choice of reference point. During surgery the operating table is often raised or lowered for the convenience of the surgeons; if the monitoring apparatus is not moved appropriately to account for this, errors will occur.

4. Changes in position of the patient will cause genuine changes in the CVP which must be taken into account when interpreting CVP trends. For instance, if the patient is moved from a horizontal to a head-down position, the CVP is likely to rise.

5. Mean intrathoracic pressure, and thereby CVP, is higher during intermittent positive pressure ventilation than during spontaneous ventilation, making comparisons of CVP measured in a patient whose ventilation mode changes unreliable. To reduce this source of misinterpretation, it is advisable to make CVP readings at end expiration, where, in the majority of patients, the intrathoracic pressures in the two ventilation modes are

comparable. The CVP may also be affected by a thoracotomy which results in reduced intrathoracic pressure during intermittent positive pressure ventilation.

6. CVP measurements made with water manometers are commonly quoted in centimeters of water (cm H_2O) or, more accurately, centimetres of whatever fluid has been put in the manometer. Measurements made with systems utilizing electronic pressure transducers are often in millimetres of mercury (mmHg). Care should be taken to account for these different units if the patient is transferred from one monitoring system to another. The conversion is:

$$1 \text{ cm } H_2O = 1.36 \text{ mmHg}$$

7. Short-term variations in CVP can be produced by surgical obstruction to venous return, e.g. inferior vena caval compression during laparotomy, by tying an internal jugular vein during a neck dissection, and by coughing or straining.

Physiological significance

There are three factors which determine the CVP.

Venous capacitance

If other factors are unchanged, an increase in overall venous tone will decrease the venous capacitance and therefore increase the CVP and vice versa.

Intravascular volume

An increase in intravascular blood volume will be reflected by an increase in CVP, and vice versa, if other factors are unchanged.

43

Cardiac function

In the absence of changes in venous capacitance and intravascular volume, a rise in CVP indicates a deterioration in cardiac function. If the CVP is initially high, and then falls, this is indicative of improving cardiac function.

Aetiology

Venous capacitance

Venous tone, and hence venous capacitance, can be affected by direct pharmacological and neurally mediated factors. Veins are seldom affected in isolation, and in general, venodilation or venoconstriction is a part of vasodilation or vasoconstriction.
Direct pharmacological factors. Venodilators include most anaesthetic agents, antihypertensive drugs with a direct vasodilator action (especially nitrates), and some sedative and tranquillizing drugs, notably the phenothiazines and butyrophenones. Venoconstrictors include alpha-adrenoceptor agonists and beta-antagonists.
Neurally mediated factors. Sympathetic fibres innervate the vascular system, so that agents which modulate central sympathetic output or the conduction of afferent traffic will affect venous tone.

Central – Most anaesthetic agents will reduce overall sympathetic activity, with the exception of ketamine and cyclopropane. Sedative and analgesic agents have a qualitatively similar action. Some antihypertensive drugs, e.g. clonidine, possess a central sympatholytic action in the absence of global cerebral depression. Surgical stimulus, unless the patient is deeply anaesthetized or completely pain-free, will increase sympathetic activity, as will fear and anxiety in the awake patient. An increase in venous tone is a physiological response to hypovolaemia mediated by the sympathetic nervous system. Hypothermia and hypocarbia have a vasoconstricting effect.

Peripheral – Surgical or chemical sympathectomy will reduce venous tone, as will the sympathectomy associated with reversible nerve blocks, notably spinal and epidural anaesthesia. Indirectly or directly acting sympathomimetics, alpha-receptor agonists and beta-antagonists will increase venous tone.

Intravascular volume

A drop in intravascular volume may be due to loss of blood or a reduction in plasma volume. Blood loss during surgery is usually evident; however, its extent may be underestimated due to inaccurate assessment in weighing swabs and measuring suction losses, or by concealed loss under surgical drapes or on to the floor. Occult loss of large volumes of blood may also occur, and should always be considered, particularly in traumatized patients who may have undiagnosed sources of haemorrhage. Occult loss is often into closed body compartments, and includes haemothorax, haemoperitoneum, bleeds into the gut, lung contusion, bleeds into extensively injured muscle and around fractures of long bones.

Reduction of plasma volume may be due to fluid loss into the 'third space', i.e. the extracellular space, and occurs particularly in patients with bowel obstruction and during laparotomies which involve extensive gut exposure and handling. Traumatized tissue, and especially that suffering from burn injury, can deprive the circulation of fluid in a similar manner. Evaporative loss is common in operations where the chest or abdomen is open, or with large areas of skin loss. Such loss is accentuated in a pyrexial patient. All urine is derived from the intravascular compartment, and a large diuresis may account for significant losses in volume. Loss of water vapour by exhalation is accentuated in patients ventilated with dry gases. All these losses become more significant during prolonged surgery.

An increase in intravascular volume is most commonly

caused by iatrogenic intravenous infusion. Notable exceptions to this include absorption of fluid from the prostatic bed during transurethral resection and through the peritoneum and pleura after 'wash-outs'. The amount absorbed in this way is proportional to the time of exposure and is therefore likely to be more significant in prolonged operations.

Cardiac function

A rise in CVP, usually associated with a fall in blood pressure, is seen during periods of deterioration in cardiac function. More accurately, it is suggestive of right heart failure. It cannot, however, be specified from the rise in CVP whether this is primary right heart failure, or that subsequent to left heart failure or extracardiac causes such as cardiac tamponade and pulmonary embolism. If further diagnostic data are required in this respect, it may be desirable to measure left atrial pressure or pulmonary capillary wedge pressure. It is beyond the scope of this chapter to delineate all the factors that are operative in producing heart failure; however, the following list gives some of those factors that may be encountered during anaesthesia.

1. *Decreased contractility due to myocardial ischaemia*: the occurrence of myocardial ischaemia is determined by the balance between oxygen supply and myocardial oxygen demand. Oxygen supply will be compromised by hypotension, arrhythmias, tachycardia, hypoxia, coronary artery occlusion, stenosis or spasm and profound anaemia. Myocardial oxygen demand will be increased by hypertension, tachycardia, overtransfusion, increased blood viscosity, increased peripheral vascular resistance and valvular malfunction.
2. *Other causes of decreased contractility*: these include acidosis, hypothermia, parasympathetic stimulation and drug effects such as beta-adrenergic blocking drugs, cal-

46

cium channel blockers and withdrawal of catecholamines. Most general and local anaesthetic agents are negative inotropes.

3. *Increased afterload*: an increase in peripheral vascular resistance, whether due to physiological and pharmacological factors, or to physical obstruction such as aortic clamping, may cause a deterioration in cardiac function.

4. *Increased preload*: abnormally high CVP will, of itself, adversely affect cardiac function by overstretching the myocardium.

5. *Rate and rhythm effects*: the cardiac output is the product of the stroke volume and the heart rate. Severe bradycardia will produce a low-output situation by its reduction of the heart rate, while extreme tachycardia may reduce stroke volume by allowing inadequate time for ventricular filling. The loss of the atrial adjunct to ventricular filling may, in certain patients with borderline cardiac function, significantly reduce cardiac output, and therefore rhythm changes away from normal sinus rhythm may initiate heart failure.

Improvement in cardiac function from a previously suboptimal situation may lower the CVP and may result from correction of reversible factors initiating the deterioration, sympathetic stimulation, parasympathetic inhibition and the administration of positive inotropic drugs such as dopamine, dobutamine, adrenalin, etc.

Management

The monitoring of the CVP should be considered as a useful adjunct to the monitoring of other physiological parameters during anaesthetic practice. Careful consideration of the patient's preoperative condition, blood pressure, heart rate and rhythym, temperature, peripheral perfusion, ventilation and oxygenation, anaesthetic depth, urine output, drug therapy, etc. must be taken into account before management decisions are made. Having made a diagnosis aided by information derived from CVP readings, the effectiveness of management interventions should be assessed not only by the response in the CVP, but also by that of other parameters monitored.

In simple terms, CVP monitoring is normally used in anaesthetic practice for the following reasons:

1. To help differentiate between hypovolaemia and cardiac failure as causes of hypotension.
2. To assess the efficacy of treatment aimed at replacing volume loss and correcting cardiac failure.
3. As a guide to the adequacy of volume replacement during surgical procedures in which large blood losses or fluid shifts are expected.
4. To assist the monitoring of patients at risk from cardiac decompensation during anaesthesia.

Provided that the causes of spurious variations in CVP are excluded, and changes in venous capacitance are taken into account, CVP measurement can be very useful in the above situations. One should beware, however, of acting on a single absolute reading. Most often it is the trend in the CVP that produces useful information during anaesthesia.

The management of changes in CVP due to variation in intravascular volume are usually straightforward: the hypovolaemic patient should be given intravenous fluid of an appropriate variety; care should be taken not to overtransfuse the patient. Incipient overtransfusion can often be identified when the CVP, which has been rising gradually during a steady infusion, begins to rise more rapidly. Infusion should be withheld from the hypervolaemic patient, and in severe cases, venesection may be considered, whether physical or pharmacological, with the use of vasodilators.

CVP rises due to deteriorating cardiac function should

initiate a search for the cause of the deterioration. If an easily reversible cause is found, appropriate action should be taken. If this is not the case, the use of inotropic agents should be considered. CVP falls due to improving cardiac function may be welcome, but in themselves do not indicate a need for treatment.

Hypotension during regional anaesthesia

Definition

Hypotension is a common complication of spinal (subarachnoid and epidural) anaesthesia. It may be defined as a fall in the mean arterial pressure of 30 per cent of the resting value. Whereas a reduction in blood pressure of this magnitude may have few physiological implications in young healthy individuals, it may have devastating effects in patients with cardiovascular and cerebrovascular disease; it is important to bear this variation in mind when considering therapeutic intervention if a fall in blood pressure does occur.

Hypotension in obstetric patients may be defined in a more scientific fashion. No autoregulatory mechanisms exist in uterine blood vessels and therefore flow in these vessels is dependent solely on maternal blood pressure. It has been suggested that a fall in systolic blood pressure to below 90 mmHg may result in a sufficient reduction in uteroplacental flow to produce fetal bradycardia and acidosis. It would seem reasonable, therefore to define hypotension in obstetric patients as a fall in systolic pressure to below this level.

Diagnosis

Diagnosis depends on regular monitoring and recording of blood pressure. A close rapport with the patient is also essential; subjective feelings such as faintness or nausea may indicate a fall in cerebral perfusion and alert the anaesthetist to the possibility of a low blood pressure. If the hypotension is of sufficient degree to affect the cerebral blood flow it must be corrected.

Aetiology

A number of mechanisms operate during spinal anaesthesia to produce a fall in blood pressure. Preganglionic sympathetic B fibres are blocked early, producing vasodilation with consequent pooling of blood. This, in turn, leads to a decreased venous return and cardiac output. Although some compensation for this fall occurs by a reflex increase in vasoconstrictor activity in the arms, the overall effect is a decrease in the cardiac output.

If the spinal block extends to the T5–T_2 level, blockade of splanchnic nerves will result in pooling of blood in the gut, and this will further decrease venous return. At this level of blockade, catecholamine secretion from the adrenal medulla is also reduced with consequent decreases in heart rate and cardiac output. If the block reaches T1–T4, cardiac sympathetic reflexes are abolished with decreased chronotropic and inotropic drive. The vagal predominance which ensues may manifest itself as a sudden bradycardia or even vagal arrest. Moreover, at this level of blockade, the compensatory vasoconstriction in the upper half of the body is lost; venous return and cardiac output will fall further.

When considering the pregnant patient, the important factor of inferior vena caval occlusion must be borne in mind. Occlusion of the vena cava by the uterus occurs in most pregnant women when in the supine position. Normally the resulting falls in venous return and cardiac output are compensated for by lower limb vasoconstriction, and by shunting of venous blood through the paravertebral plexus. However, this compensation is ineffective in the presence of spinal blockade; in this situation the fall in blood pressure may be precipitous and profound. It is therefore essential that women in the later weeks of pregnancy undergoing spinal anaesthesia should be placed in the left lateral position by the use of a wedge under their backs.

Other factors may contribute to or exacerbate a fall in blood pressure during spinal anaesthesia. Untreated hypovolaemia may cause profound hypotension when the block is instituted. Absorption of local anaesthetic agent into the systemic circulation may also influence blood pressure. Whilst low blood levels of these agents may have minimal effects on the cardiovascular system, toxic levels cause decreased myocardial contractility and vascular dilation. These effects will be more profound if convulsions occur and hypoxia intervenes. Concomitant treatment with certain drugs (e.g. beta-adrenergic blocking drugs, vasodilators) may also increase the occurrence of hypotension during spinal anaesthesia.

Physiological significance

Maintenance of perfusion of vital organs requires an adequate blood pressure. When moderate falls in blood pressure occur, autoregulatory mechanisms intervene and allow preservation of tissue flow. However, if the blood pressure is allowed to fall further, there comes a point when these compensatory mechanisms cannot cope, and blood flow will fall. The point at which this occurs varies from individual to individual. For example, a young healthy patient may well tolerate a systolic blood pressure of 70 mmHg; in contrast, the same pressure in an elderly patient with ischaemic heart disease may severely compromise coronary artery blood flow and result in myocardial ischaemia. It is essential, therefore, that the anaesthetist should fully assess the cardiovascular, cerebral and renal function of each patient when considering spinal anaesthesia and when deciding when to intervene to correct any ensuing hypotension.

Management

Although common, hypotension during spinal anaesthesia is by no means unavoidable. Thorough assessment of each patient should be carried out before performing the block and this should include a full drug history. At this stage, it is wise to decide on the degree of fall of blood pressure that is permissible before intervention is necessary. Immediately prior to establishing the block, the patient should be preloaded with a balanced electrolyte solution or colloid. Depending on the cardiovascular status of the patient, a volume equivalent to 10–20 per cent of the circulating blood volume should be administered if more than five vertebral segments are to be blocked. The choice of fluid does not appear to be critical. Women in the late stages of pregnancy should be managed in the left lateral position.

Before administration of the local anaesthetic agent, it is essential to aspirate on the needle or catheter, thus minimizing the possibility of inadvertent intravascular injection. The agent should be injected slowly.

If, despite these measures, an unacceptable fall in blood pressure does occur, additional intravenous fluid should be given and the patient placed in the Trendelenburg position (care should be exercised if the patient has been given a subarachnoid injection of a hyperbaric local anaesthetic solution as the head-down position may encourage further rostral spread). Oxygen should be administered via a facemask. If the blood pressure fails to rise following these manoeuvres, a vasopressor agent should be given. Ephedrine (5–15 mg intravenously) is the agent most commonly favoured, especially for the pregnant patient, as although the drug does cross the placenta, it appears to restore maternal blood pressure without significantly decreasing uterine blood flow.

The difficult airway

To the experienced anaesthetist there are many indications which give warning of possible difficulties in maintaining an airway in a particular patient.

The most obvious is gross facial deformity such as Treacher Collins syndrome or a patient with facial distortions due to disease or trauma. Less obvious is the patient with a poorly developed mandible which restricts the room available in the oropharynx to accommodate the tongue (Fig. 2.1). The patient with a short distance between the hyoid and the mandible

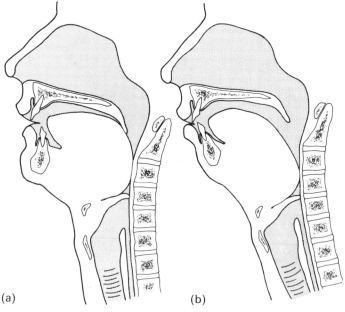

(a)　　　　　　　　　　　　　　　　(b)

Fig. 2.1 (a) Normal anatomy
(b) Effect of an underslung lower jaw with a poorly developed mandible.

might be difficult to ventilate and intubate. The bull-necked, the obese, the arthritic, those with rheumatoid disease of the vertebrae and arytenoids in patients with ankylosing spondylitis and those with gross dental deformity may all present problems.

Once the possibility has arisen that maintenance of the airway is likely to be difficult, it is sensible to take precautions to minimize or eliminate these problems. If, however, the patient is anaesthetized and in spite of respiratory effort on his or her part there is little or no gas exchange it is necessary to analyse the problem and correct the situation urgently.

WHERE IS THE DIFFICULTY?

Laryngeal level

This should be suspected if there is no gas exchange in spite of violent patient effort during inspiration, associated with crowing inspiratory noises and unrelieved by elevating the mandible. Laryngeal spasm is common if an irritant volatile agent is introduced too suddenly into the gas mixture – try turning it off. It may result from mucus or saliva irritating the cords. A quick gentle suck with a soft catheter will clear away offending material, as may the simple manoeuvre of head-down tilt.

An artificial airway introduced in too light a plane of anaesthesia is a common provoking factor – remove the airway.

Once these remedies have been carried out, positive end-expiratory pressure applied using a distended reservoir bag full of oxygen encourages what little gas exchange is taking place. Do not screw the Heidbrink valve completely down in this situation to avoid the generation of too high a pressure. If in spite of these remedies the patient does not open the glottis, seek help. If help is not available and the diagnosis is assured, a small dose of suxamethonium may be used to break the laryngeal spasm.

Tongue level

This is due to inability to maintain a patent posterior oropharynx when the mandible is elevated due to a disproportionately enlarged tongue or a small mandible. In patients with small or absent mandibles the relatively bulky tongue results in the epiglottis being pushed backwards, so that it acts as a flap to cover the laryngeal orifice. In extreme conditions when an oropharyngeal airway does not relieve the condition, a nasopharyngeal airway may help. If this does not relieve the obstruction a tongue clip placed in the dorsum of the tongue and used to pull it forward is a drastic but potentially life-saving method of opening up the oropharynx. This manoeuvre not only pulls the tongue away from the posterior pharyngeal wall but also elevates the epiglottis so that it no longer flaps over the larynx. Alternative airways, such as the Brain laryngeal mask or Portex cuffed nasopharyngeal tube (Fig. 2.2) may be used.

Other lesser problems that may be encountered include the difficulties of obtaining a good fit with a facemask due to facial deformities – this problem can usually be overcome with the help of swabs to pad out the defects and a high gas flow. Patients with trismus or ankylosis of the temporomandibular joints require very careful assessment.

The possible combinations of circumstances that might cause difficulty in maintaining an airway are legion. Certain principles apply to all:

1. If the difficulty is such that oxygenation is not possible, seek assistance or abandon the procedure. A disappointed patient is better than a dead one!

2. Never take away the patient's powers of spontaneous ventilation without first assuring oneself that intermittent positive pressure ventilation is possible. Once the patient is asleep it is usually possible to establish whether or not it will be feasible to ventilate him or her following the

administration of a muscle relaxant by assisting the patient's spontaneous inspiratory efforts by squeezing the reservoir bag during inspiration.

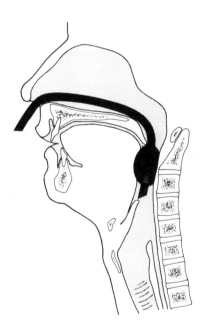

Fig. 2.2 Use of the Portex cuffed nasopharyngeal tube used to overcome a difficult airway problem

Difficult intubation

Definition

A difficult intubation lies somewhere between an easy intubation and an impossible one. Although this may sound trite, it is
a reasonable definition for a situation commonly met in
anaesthetic practice. It implies that, provided ideal circumstances can be produced, intubation is possible by skilled
intervention.

Diagnosis

Like the difficult airway, experience allows one to recognize
some of the indications of possible problems in advance. Once
one has embarked upon the intubation, its difficulty becomes
apparent, although occasionally it may not manifest itself until
repeated oesophageal intubations have been produced.

Significance

Trauma to the airway may cause bruising, haemorrhage,
contamination of the airway, or oedema which may dangerously narrow or even occlude the airway, making ventilation
difficult or impossible. Even if such trauma does not present
danger to the patient, it may cause considerable postoperative
discomfort. Enthusiastic attempts at a difficult intubation may
dislodge or break teeth, cut lips, cause haemorrhage into the
uvula and damage the palate. Tears in the pharyngeal mucosa
have been reported, including penetration of the pyriform
fossa. The greater the pharyngeal trauma, the more difficult is
subsequent intubation. It is therefore important not to persist
to a point where a difficult intubation has produced conditions
which make intubation impossible.

If the patient has a full stomach, protracted attempts at
intubation increase the period in which the airway is unpro-
tected, and therefore at risk from contamination.

Preoccupation with attempts at intubation may cause inattention to other important aspects of anaesthetic care, viz. oxygenation and amnesia, with the result that the patient may become hypoxic or start to wake up.

Delay of surgery, even if only by a few minutes, may in certain circumstances considerably increase the risk to the patient. Hypoxia and hypercarbia combined with light anaesthesia may cause a rise in blood pressure and increase hypoxia, thus considerably increasing the risk to some patients. Trauma to the vocal cords and larynx may make the patient difficult to settle and increase the risk of him or her straining once the tube is in place. For all these reasons it is important to seek assistance or abandon the intubation if medically feasible before conditions deteriorate.

Aetiology

Much stress is placed on the anatomical variations or pathological afflictions of the patient. However, other factors may contribute to produce a difficult intubation.

Intubator

The greater the experience the lower will be the incidence of difficulty with intubations.

Situation

The difficulty may be greater if it is not carried out in an operating theatre environment in the presence of trained assistance.

Equipment

A functioning laryngoscope and an endotracheal tube are all that is required for the vast majority of intubations. However, some more difficult situations may require additional equipment to make them easy, or indeed, possible. These include good lighting, suction, gum elastic bougies, fibreoptic laryngoscopes, a selection of endotracheal tubes etc.

Technique

It is too often presumed that the easiest approach to the larynx is by direct visualization made possible with a laryngoscope. Whilst this is usually true, there are some patients who present a difficult oral intubation and who may be easily intubated with a blind nasal technique.

Anaesthetic

The anaesthetic being employed may be inappropriate for the technique of intubation being attempted. The conduct of a rapid-sequence induction ('crash' induction) may lead the anaesthetist to attempt induction before the patient is fully relaxed.

Difficulty in intubation can often be predicted prior to

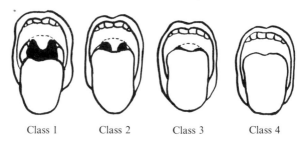

Class 1   Class 2   Class 3   Class 4

Fig. 2.3 An assessment scheme to aid the prediction of difficult intubations. The structures seen when the patients open their mouths fully and protrude their tongue to a maximum.

Class 1: Soft palate, fauces, uvula, pillars
Class 2: Soft palate, fauces, uvula
Class 3: Soft palate, base of uvula
Class 4: Soft palate not visible

Given normal laryngeal anatomy, patients in Class 1 and 2 should provide little difficulty in intubation. Patients in Class 3, and particularly those in Class 4, may provide difficulty in intubation.
After: Mallampati SR (1983). Clinical signs to predict difficult tracheal intubation (hypothesis). Can. Anaesth. Soc. J. 30, 316–7.

Illustration from: Samsoon GLT, Young JRB (1987). Difficult tracheal intubation: a retrospective study *Anaesthesia 42*, 487–490.

anaesthesia. Preoperative assessment schemes exist which may assist such prediction (Fig. 2.3). However, there remains a minority in whom it is not possible to anticipate difficulty before an intubation attempt is made. This is usually due to a combination of minor anatomical variations or an unexpected pathological finding. If difficult intubation is anticipated help should be obtained before starting the anaesthetic and under no circumstances should the patient be paralysed unless it can first be demonstrated that artificial ventilation is possible.

Management

In all circumstances the prime factor of importance is the maintenance of adequate oxygenation. Attention should also be paid to anaesthesia and, if necessary, relaxation. The following points should be considered.

Does the patient need to be intubated?

Can the procedure be carried out safely using a bag and mask? There is an increasing trend for intubation to be performed for convenience rather than necessity. Having appreciated the difficulty of an intubation, it is not inappropriate, in the interests of the patient, to abandon intubation for a technique which includes maintenance of the airway by another means, provided that the patient is not thereby exposed to unnecessary risk. The use of a laryngeal mask or a cuffed nasotracheal airway may suffice and obviate the need for intubation of the larynx.

Should a more experienced anaesthetist be called?

Should the patient be allowed to wake up?

Should another technique that avoids intubation be used, i.e. a local block?

Is there an easier technique of intubation for this patient?

It is reasonable to persist in attempts at intubation for a short period provided that the patient is continuing to be well oxygenated and asleep.

These efforts may be assisted by backwards displacement of the larynx by an assistant during laryngoscopy, by the use of a malleable soft bougie as an introducer (great care must be exercised if a bougie is used lest the pyriform fossa or retropharyngeal tissues be perforated). Blind nasal intubation with the patient breathing spontaneously, or under full muscle relaxation, often succeeds where oral intubation fails. The technique of blind nasal intubation is made easier by allowing the patient to breath 5–10 per cent carbon dioxide so that he or she hyperventilates and opens the glottic aperture to its maximum capacity before intubation is attempted during inspiration.

The use of a fibreoptic laryngoscope to guide intubation may be effective, but is often less successful when used after failed laryngoscopic intubation as blood and mucus in the oropharynx obscure the operator's vision. It is therefore better to use this as an elective technique, with the patient awake and sedated.

Confirmation of the position of an endotracheal tube

The only foolproof method of determining the position of the endotracheal tube is by passing a fibreoptic bronchoscope through its lumen and observing the rings of the trachea and the carina. In extreme cases this manoeuvre should be carried out.

Capnography is a useful tool for checking tube position. Although expired air blown into the stomach by bag and mask ventilation prior to intubation may give rise to carbon dioxide being detected after oesophageal intubation, the effect is short-lived and the continued presence of carbon dioxide in expired gas strongly suggests that the tube is in the trachea.

DIFFICULT INTUBATION

All other methods of determining endotracheal location of the tube may at times give false assurance:

1. Visualization of the tube passing between the cords as it enters the larynx (tubes can concertina and spring back into the oesophagus).

2. Observation of chest movement between the nipples and the clavicles.

3. Auscultation of the chest and hearing vesicular breath sounds on inflating the lungs (this is the same physical sign as above, but using a different monitor – ears rather than eyes – and it is not foolproof).

4. Auscultation over the stomach – the presence of bubbling sounds on inflation suggests that the tube is in the wrong place. However, absence of these sounds does not confirm the correct position.

5. Feeling the cuff in the trachea by palpation in the suprasternal notch during rapid cuff inflation. This is also a useful confirmatory sign that the tube is not too long.

Management of difficulties encountered: oral intubation

Difficulty inserting the laryngoscope

1. Ensure adequate relaxation.
2. Further extend the head if possible.
3. If cricoid pressure is being applied, ensure the assistant's fingers are not obstructing insertion.
4. Rotate laryngoscope 90° so that the handle points towards the patient's ear. Insert and rotate back to 0°.
5. Detach handle from blade, insert blade, re-attach handle.
6. Consider using Polio blade or Yentis attachment.

Difficulty visualizing larynx

1. Ensure adequate relaxation.
2. Ensure adequate neck flexion and atlanto-occipital extension.
3. Ask assistant to push larynx posteriorly. If this is already being done, ask assistant to move larynx laterally in case the larynx has been displaced in this plane.
4. Consider use of different laryngoscope, i.e. a larger one or one of different design.

Difficulty intubating an anterior larynx

1. Select a tube which is more curved.
2. Insert a malleable bougie introducer to provide adequate curvature.
3. Intubate with a gum elastic bougie, railroad tube over this.

If tube will pass through cords, but no further

1. Try a smaller tube.

Management of difficulties encountered: nasal intubation

Tube passes into oesophagus

1. Ensure that head is in 'sniffing the morning air' position.
2. Ensure tube is well curved.
3. Try lifting the head off the pillow.
4. Consider using Magill's intubating forceps.
5. Consider establishing spontaneous ventilation and try again, using carbon dioxide to establish forced inspiration and maximum laryngeal orifice.

If tube passes through cords, but no further

1. Lift the head well up to flex the neck.
2. Use a smaller tube.

If tube ends in one pyriform fossa

1. Rotate the head to same side or tube to opposite side.
2. Try the other nostril.

Other techniques

If the above manoeuvres fail, it may be reasonable or necessary to consider other techniques of intubation. These include the use of a fibreoptic bronchoscope and a Flexi-Lum inserted through an endotracheal tube. This will transilluminate the larynx, allowing the tip of the Flexi-Lum and the tube to be guided into the laryngeal orifice.

A guide wire or an epidural catheter can be passed retrogradely through the cricothyroid membrane, picked up in the oropharynx, and used to railroad the tube into the larynx. Tracheotomy or cricothyrotomy can be employed. We do not recommend that junior anaesthetists attempt these techniques without adequate supervision and instruction, except in the most dire emergency.

Postscript

If difficulty is experienced intubating a patient's trachea, make a clear note on the anaesthetic record describing the difficulty encountered and how it was solved. The knowledge will be valuable for anaesthetists managing the patient in the future. If you feel that the patient will pose a problem for any anaesthetist in the future, consider adorning the cover of the patient's notes with the words '*difficult intubation*', and making reference to the enclosed anaesthetic record. One may consider telling the patient about the difficulties encountered, or giving him or her a letter to give to any anaesthetist describing the problem. Some departments even recommend that such patients are given Medic-Alert bracelets.

Failed intubation

Definition

If a difficult intubation lies somewhere between an easy intubation and an impossible intubation, it should not be presumed that a failed intubation is synonymous with an impossible intubation. A failed intubation is a management decision made when it is felt that persistence with attempts at intubation would not be in the interest of the patient, and a management plan which does not include intubation at that time must be made.

Significance

A mismanaged failed intubation can kill. The cause of death in such a situation is almost invariably hypoxia. The anaesthetist must appreciate that the first priority is to ensure that the patient is well oxygenated. Intubation itself must take second place to this. It should be remembered that few patients will die if they are not intubated whereas all patients will die if they are not given oxygen.

Management

The important concepts involved in the management of the potential failed intubation situation are outlined in the algorithm (Fig. 2.4) and accompanying notes.

1. See 'Difficult intubation', p. 60.
2. See 'Difficult Airway', p. 56.
3. This is termed a 'danger area' as the cycle of repeated attempts at intubation while the patient becomes more hypoxic and the anaesthetist creates more trauma to the airway is one that results in significant morbidity and

PROBLEMS IN ANAESTHESIA

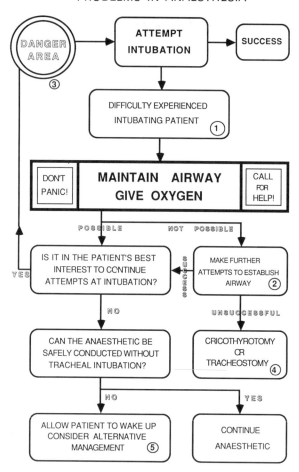

Fig. 2.4 An algorithm for the management of difficult and failed intubation.

mortality. We recommend that, except in exceptional circumstances, this route should not be travelled more than once by the anaesthetist in training.

4. The number of patients who will need cricothyrotomy or tracheostomy as a life-saving procedure is very, very small. Usually, in this situation, the use of oral or nasopharyngeal airways, adjustments to head and jaw position, alterations in depth of anaesthesia and relaxation, etc. will produce an adequate airway for oxygenation.

5. Such alternative management may include the use of local or regional anaesthesia, awake intubation or different approaches to or techniques of intubation. Management at this stage must be discussed with an experienced anaesthetist.

Difficulty in ventilation

Definition

Assuming that the anaesthetic apparatus is functioning properly, there are times when, following endotracheal intubation, or even during an otherwise uneventful anaesthetic, the inflation pressure rises or the machine fails adequately to inflate the lungs in spite of adequate muscle relaxation.

Physiological significance

Depending on the ventilation system in use, an increase in the breathing circuit, endotracheal tube or airways resistance, or a reduction in lung or chest wall compliance will cause an increase in inflation pressure, a reduction in minute ventilation, or both. High inflation pressure in the trachea may give rise to barotrauma such as pneumothorax and mucosal damage. Low minute ventilation may give rise to hypercarbia and hypoxia.

Diagnosis and management

In cases of difficulty when mechanically ventilating a patient one should change to manual ventilation. This may identify the source of difficulty as being the mechanical ventilation system itself. If significant resistance to ventilation continues, briefly disconnect the circuit at the tube connector and inflate. This excludes malfunction of the manual ventilation system and implies that the cause of difficulty in ventilation is distal to the endotracheal tube connector. It is commonly held that manually ventilating the patient in this instance gives one a greater appreciation of the degree of resistance to ventilation.

Tracheal tube obstruction can occur at any time with any type of tube. Tubes can kink (especially in the pharynx and over the teeth), can become blocked with secretions or blood, foreign bodies, or a cuff that has herniated over the end. Flexometallic latex tubes can delaminate and soften so that the cuff compresses the lumen and may kink at the junction with the connector.

A suction catheter or a gum elastic bougie should be passed through the lumen of the tracheal tube to ensure patency. Briefly deflate the cuff. If the tube is still blocked it should be removed and replaced – it is a good idea to leave the bougie in place and withdraw the tube over it in order to facilitate its replacement. The oblique end of the endotracheal tubes can be obstructed by the wall of the trachea (the Murphy Eye minimizes this risk), especially if there is a rotational distortion of the trachea during thyroidectomy or traction on the hilum of the lung.

If a double lumen endotracheal tube has been used, the patency of both lumens must be tested when the patient has been placed in position on the operating table. These tubes are most easily displaced, kinked and obstructed when the patient is turned on his or her side.

Pulmonary causes of failure to ventilate include secretions or blood blocking an airway, surgical interference, pneumo- or haemothorax and bronchospasm. The latter, if severe, is a frightening condition that needs energetic treatment (see p. 81). The onset of pulmonary oedema and pulmonary interstitial oedema may simulate bronchospasm as compliance is increased and expiratory wheezes may be heard.

Although many different causes of difficulty in ventilation have been described, we would strongly recommend that if ventilation becomes extremely difficult, and if effective ventilation cannot be rapidly restored, the problem should be presumed to lie with the tracheal tube. It should be removed, and ventilation with bag and mask should continue until a new tube can be checked and replaced in the trachea. Only once this has been done can alterations in ventilation (e.g. increasing inflation pressure, reducing tidal volume) be made, while a remediable cause for the difficulty in ventilation is sought and corrected.

Laryngospasm

Definition

Laryngospasm may be defined as partial or absolute obstruction of the glottis by the action of the intrinsic laryngeal muscles. However, in the clinical setting it is often difficult to differentiate true laryngospasm from disorders that give rise to airway obstruction at the glottic level, and these will be included within our discussion of laryngospasm.

Diagnosis

True laryngospasm in the normal patient is the product of light planes of anaesthesia associated with a stimulus (usually to the pharynx or larynx), which combine to trigger the protective reflexes of the larynx in an exaggerated form. Laryngospasm may be mimicked by obstruction of the glottis for other reasons, e.g. oedema, foreign body and tumours.

The problem identified by the anaesthetist is that of significant resistance to gas flow, and the presumption that the source of resistance is the glottis is reached by confirming the normal function of the anaesthetic circuit and the maintenance of a clear pharyngeal airway by holding the jaw well forward and inserting an oral or nasopharyngeal airway. These manoeuvres in fact identify the resistance as occurring at the glottis or below, and the identification of laryngospasm is usually completed by the finding of absolute obstruction to gas flow to the lungs, or the association of high resistance to gas flow with crowing or grunting noises from the larynx. The passage of a gas through a narrow orifice at high speed sets up turbulence, and in the case of laryngospasm, this turbulence of gas flow causes the vocal cords to vibrate, giving rise to crowing noises.

Laryngospasm cannot be diagnosed in the presence of a correctly placed tracheal tube.

Physiological significance

Inadequate ventilation of the patient will cause hypoxia and hypercarbia. This is associated with excessive muscular effort by the patient, increasing his or her oxygen demand.

Enthusiastic attempts at intermittent positive pressure ventilation with a circuit and mask in the presence of a closed glottis may inflate the stomach, and encourage regurgitation of stomach contents.

Spontaneous ventilation by the patient against a closed glottis may cause high negative intrathoracic pressures, which have been associated with the development of pulmonary oedema.

Aetiology

True laryngospasm

Laryngospasm may occur during induction of anaesthesia where inadequate anaesthesia is combined with a stimulus to the airway. This is especially true if an attempt is made to deepen light anaesthesia too quickly using either isoflurane or enflurane in high concentrations, as their vapour is pungent and irritant. It may be caused by other irritants to the airway, e.g. secretions, blood, vomitus, insertion of airways, positive pressure ventilation and attempts at laryngoscopy. Barbiturates are said to increase airway sensitivity at light planes of anaesthesia. Children are thought to be more prone to laryngospasm than adults, especially at the end of operations following extubation of the trachea.

During maintenance of anaesthesia, laryngospasm may occur in the presence of the above stimulae, or with a powerful surgical stimulus if the patient is not deeply anaesthetized. This occurs commonly during anal stretch and dilation of the cervix, though it may happen in association with any painful surgical stimulus.

LARYNGOSPASM

Light planes of anaesthesia are inevitable during emergence. The stimulus to laryngospasm is often that of extubation, and for this reason the old axiom 'extubate deep or awake, but never in between' arose. Laryngospasm triggered by the presence of secretions or blood is more likely to occur if the patient is not placed in a position that encourages drainage away from the larynx. Extubation spasm is more readily produced in hypoxic patients. It is sensible therefore to ensure ventilation with high inspired oxygen before it is carried out.

Glottic obstruction for other reasons

Oedema of the vocal cords or other glottic structures can closely mimick laryngospasm. Causes include:

Laryngeal or pharyngeal infection, inflammation or trauma
Prolonged endotracheal intubation (for days rather than hours)
Use of relatively large endotracheal tube, e.g. in the very young, or after the use of double lumen endobronchial tubes
Repeated attempts at intubation
Surgery to the larynx, neck and thyroid
Prolonged raised venous pressure, e.g. head-down position, superior vena caval occlusion
As part of a drug reaction
Radiotherapy

The glottis may also be obstructed by:

Foreign bodies, notably thick secretions, blood clots, teeth, throat packs, and items of anaesthetic or surgical equipment
Bilateral recurrent laryngeal nerve palsy, usually associated with surgery to the neck
Tumours
Causes external to the larynx, e.g. haematoma or swelling in the neck. This usually starts as bleeding below the mylo-

hyoid and tracks downwards in tissue planes to cause supraglottic and glottic oedema. If it occurs following infection and abscess formation it causes Ludwig's angina – a surgical emergency.

Management

The aim of management is to ensure adequate oxygenation of the patient while taking steps to relieve the laryngospasm or other remediable causes of glottic obstruction. The anaesthetist must, as ever, observe and monitor the patient closely.

Give oxygen in concentrations up to 100 per cent bearing in mind that during induction and maintenance of anaesthesia the withdrawal of nitrous oxide may further lighten anaesthesia and worsen the situation.

Deepen anaesthesia by the administration of an intravenous anaesthetic. As the patient is hypoventilating, administration of higher concentrations of inhalational anaesthetic is unlikely to be successful. Some anaesthetists give intravenous lignocaine (up to 1.5 mg/kg) to reduce airway sensitivity.

Ensure airway is free of secretions by suctioning (under direct vision if feasible).

Consider positive pressure ventilation. If the above manoeuvres are unsuccessful, if the patient is at risk from becoming hypoxic, or if he or she is apnoeic, gentle intermittent positive pressure ventilation may assist oxygenation. If the patient is attempting spontaneous ventilation, try to time ventilation with inspiratory efforts. Some authorities recommend positive pressure during expiration as well i.e. continuous positive airway pressure.

Consider use of muscle relaxants. If the patient is still obstructed and it is certain that muscle spasm is the cause, it may be necessary to 'break' the laryngospasm by paralysing the laryngeal muscles. A small dose of suxamethonium (1 mg/kg) is usually all that is needed. The patient will need positive pressure ventilation once this has been given, but if oxygenation allows, insert a laryngoscope to allow direct visualization of the larynx and removal of secretions, vomitus or foreign bodies. The use of suxamethonium does not necessarily imply the need for intubation. If the airway is clear, the larynx normal, and intubation is not required for the conduct of the anaesthetic, deepen the patient with inhalational agents and await the return of spontaneous ventilation. Extreme caution must be exercised in the use of muscle relaxants in patients who have presumed or known laryngeal pathology, as ventilation may not be possible after relaxation. In this situation matters may worsen after the use of muscle relaxants. Muscle relaxants should also be used with caution in patients in whom pharyngeal soiling by blood or secretions is suspected.

The above scheme and the timing of the above steps may have to be modified according to the situation, the patient's medical condition, and the likely cause of glottic obstruction. For example:

1. Glottic obstruction after extubation in a previously healthy patient who has just had a tonsillectomy. The administration of positive airway pressure by mask may be considered undesirable as there is a risk of soiling the patient's lungs with blood. Laryngoscopy and suction would be a preliminary step in management, and, if this is not possible because of masseter spasm during emergence, it may be desirable either to nurse the patient head-down or to administer suxamethonium and intubate the patient in rapid sequence before applying intermittent positive pressure ventilation.

2. Management of partial obstruction and noisy breathing in a previously normal patient who has just been extubated after a thyroidectomy may involve deepening of anaesthesia with oxygen and an inhalational agent to allow laryngoscopy and permit direct assessment of cord movement in case damage to the recurrent laryngeal nerves has been the cause of the laryngeal obstruction.

3. Laryngospasm on induction of a patient with a previous significant burn injury. The use of suxamethonium may be associated with a massive rise in serum potassium and cardiac arrest in severely burnt patients, and the anaesthetist should consider the use of a rapidly acting non-depolarizing agent if a muscle relaxant is considered necessary. This risk is greatest between 2 days and 6 months following injury. The same risk of suxamethonium-induced cardiac arrest is present in patients with recent spinal cord and crush injuries.

We strongly recommend that in managing this, and any other problem during anaesthesia, careful observation is combined with consideration of the particular problem in the particular patient, such that the management is tailored to suit the needs and safety of the individual rather than employing a rigid protocol.

Bronchospasm

Diagnosis

Bronchospasm and wheezing are not synonymous terms. Bronchospasm is only one cause of wheezing and before the diagnosis can be made, the other causes of wheezing must be excluded.

Degrees of bronchospasm exist, from mild to severe and even life-threatening. Bronchospasm causes obstruction to gas flow, and it is the consequences of respiratory obstruction that usually attract the attention of the anaesthetist. If the patient is breathing spontaneously, it may be noticed that the movements of the reservoir bag are reduced, or that the patient's chest and abdomen are moving i.e. 'see-saw' or paradoxical respiration as if he or she were obstructed. The expiratory phase may be prolonged, and accompained with active expiration using the abdominal and neck musculature. If the patient is being ventilated, it is the high inflation pressure which commonly alerts the anaesthetist to the problem. This may be accompanied by prolonged expiration as observed, or measured with a respirometer. It is uncommon for audible expiratory wheeze to be the first sign of bronchospasm, but as anaesthetic tubing can conduct and amplify such noises, this is a possibility, especially if the anaesthetist listens at the distal end of the expiratory tubing. Cyanosis may occasionally be the first sign of severe bronchospasm.

Confirmation of the diagnosis is not simply a matter of detecting wheezing on auscultation of the chest. It is equally possible to hear no wheezes in the presence of severe bronchospasm (as a result of minimal air movement), and to hear pronounced expiratory wheeze in its absence, due to turbulent airflow in tubing or apparatus. It is mainly by exclusion that confirmation is achieved. Other causes of respiratory obstruction with resultant turbulent airflow producing a wheezing noise or an increase in inflation pressure include the following.

Patient factors

Airways obstruction due to chronic disease or inspissated secretions, foreign bodies, blood clots, etc.

Obstruction to free movement of chest or abdomen by physical or surgical objects

Increase in muscular tone, i.e. coughing, straining, inadequate relaxation

Pneumothorax (particularly a tension pneumothorax), pulmonary oedema

Equipment factors

Incorrect placement of tracheal tube: oesophageal, endobronchial

Tracheal tube bevel against tracheal wall

Obstructed airway, i.e. poorly maintained airway, blocked Guedel or kinked nasopharyngeal tube or tracheal tube

Blockage, kinking of tubes or malfunction of valves in breathing/ventilating circuit

Physiological significance

Bronchospasm causes an increase in resistance to gas flow. The electrical equation $V = I \times R$ can be expressed thus: $I = V/R$, and by extension to a physiological context:

Gas flow = inflation pressure/airways resistance

To maintain the same gas flow, and hence alveolar ventilation, as the resistance increases, so must the inflation pressure. When bronchospasm is mild, this can be achieved by the spontaneously breathing patient at the expense of an increased work of breathing and raised oxygen demand or during intermittent positive pressure ventilation by increasing inflation pressure. There comes a point, however, where inflation pressure is limited by the patient's ability to achieve the necessary negative intrathoracic pressure, or where the inter-mittent positive pressure ventilation system, by virtue of the compliance of the components of the circuit, notably the reservoir bag, or by pressure-limiting valves within the system, can no longer generate the inflation pressure necessary to maintain gas flow at a level compatible with normal alveolar ventilation. At this stage, hypoventilation, and hence hyper-capnia, will occur. When the degree of bronchospasm is so severe that gas flow falls below that required to allow the amount of oxygen equal to the metabolic requirement to pass to the alveoli, hypoxia will result.

The above simple treatment ignores the role of gas flow limitation during expiration, which is a hallmark of broncho-spasm. This limits the rate of gas flow in expiration and hence alveolar minute ventilation. The natural response to the conse-quent hypoventilation is to attempt to maintain or increase inspired minute volume, causing an increase in end-expiratory lung volume, i.e. gas trapping. This further decreases the compliance of the lungs and chest wall.

The consequences of bronchospasm are therefore:

1. Increased inflation pressure, which at high pressures may cause barotrauma, including interstitial emphysema and pneumothorax.
2. Decreased alveolar ventilation, which may cause hyper-capnia leading to tachycardia, hypertension and dys-rhythmias, and eventually hypoxia and death.
3. Increased end-expiratory lung volume which causes increased inflation pressure.
4. Absolute respiratory obstruction which will give rise to hypoxia.

Aetiology

Although bronchospasm may occur in the absence of any of the aetiological factors shown in Fig. 2.5, one or more of these

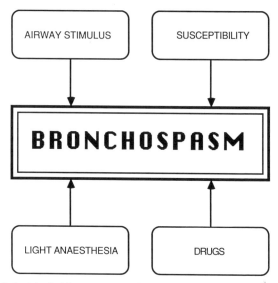

Fig. 2.5 Aetiological factors commonly operative when bronchospasm occurs

factors is commonly operative in situations where broncho-spasm occurs.

Susceptibility

Patients with a history of smoking, upper respiratory tract infection, bronchospastic disease or atopic disposition are more likely to develop bronchospasm. The anaesthetist may not be aware of such susceptibility.

Airway stimulus

The ability of the airways to respond to unwelcome invasion is limited to attempts at expulsion (coughing) and preventing the intruder from gaining access to the small airways (broncho-spasm). The degree of response, if it occurs, is proportional to the intensity of stimulus. This may range in severity from the blowing of cold dry irritant gases into the respiratory tract, through the insertion of an airway or endotracheal tube, to the placement of an endobronchial tube.

Light anaesthesia

The ability of the airway to react to invasive insults is reduced at deep levels of anaesthesia, and heightened at lighter planes of anaesthesia. Attempts to deepen light anaesthesia rapidly using irritant inhalational agents are a common cause of bronchospasm and laryngospasm.

Drugs

Certain drugs are associated with an increased incidence of bronchospasm, notably beta-adrenoceptor blocking agents and drugs which are associated with the release of histamine. Severe bronchospasm is a facet of anaphylaxis which may be initiated by anaesthetic agents (see pp. 173–175).

Management

1. Confirm the diagnosis. Exclude non-bronchospastic causes of respiratory obstruction, high inflation pressure or wheeze. Establish or continue close monitoring and observation of patient. If a particular stimulus was associated with the onset of bronchospasm, try to eliminate or reduce the stimulus if this can be done safely. Establish an unobstructed airway, even though on occasions this may seem illogical (i.e. intubating a patient who developed bronchospasm during insertion of a Guedel airway. Careful spraying of the vocal cords and trachea with local anaesthetic reduces the irritation that would otherwise result from this procedure).
2. Give oxygen. In severe bronchospasm it may be necessary to give 100 per cent oxygen to prevent hypoxia. Be

mindful that light anaesthesia in part resulting from withdrawal of nitrous oxide may worsen bronchospasm – maintain adequate anaesthesia, using intravenous agents if necessary.

3. Inhalational agents can be effective bronchodilators if the bronchospasm is not due to irritation of the airways and if minute ventilation is sufficient to allow their passage in significant concentrations to the small airways. Ether is the most effective, but is now rarely available. Halothane, enflurane and isoflurane are also effecive.

4. Phosphodiesterase inhibitors can relieve bronchospasm, but should be used cautiously. Aminophylline is usually available in anaesthetic settings. Give up to 5 mg/kg by slow intravenous injection. Rapid injection can cause dangerous dysrhythmias, particularly in the presence of hypercapnia and hypoxia.

5. Sympathomimetic agents: it is often not possible to administer these directly to the respiratory tract by aerosol in the anaesthetic setting, and so these are usually given by injection. Salbutamol 3 μg/kg or terbutaline 5 μg/kg i.v. are effective $beta_2$-adrenoceptor stimulants. If bronchospasm is severe and unrelenting, it may be necessary to use adrenalin 5–10 μg i.v. or 0.5–1 mg s.c./i.m. and repeat as necessary. All sympathomimetics may cause dangerous dysrhythmias and, especially in the presence of halothane, hypoxia and hypercarbia and the ECG should be monitored closely.

6. Other drugs: lignocaine, given intravenously in a dose of up to 1.5 mg/kg, may reduce airway reactivity and help to decrease the incidence of dysrhythmias. Ketamine has bronchodilator activity and is a non-inhalational method of maintaining anaesthesia; however, hypertension, tachycardia and emergence phenomena limit its use. Steroids and antihistamine agents have been advocated in this context; however, they are unlikely to be effective during the time course of the acute problem.

BRONCHOSPASM

Consideration should be given to the mode of ventilation. A spontaneously breathing patient is unlikely to be able to maintain adequate gas exchange in the face of moderate to severe bronchospasm. It may be necessary to convert to intermittent positive pressure ventilation. Allowing a long expiratory time during intermittent positive pressure ventilation will allow better emptying of the lungs. A longer inflation time will limit inflation pressure. However, there comes a point when prolonged inflation and expiration times will limit minute ventilation, and compromises will have to be made. The ventilation system may not be able to deal with the high inflation pressures necessary, and a different system may have to be used.

Severe bronchospasm is a frightening occurrence. Although not always predictable, if it is detected and treated early the vicious circle of increased oxygen demand by the body, producing rapid early hypoxia and hypercarbia which aggravates the bronchospasm can be broken. It should always be borne in mind that the one drug that is life-saving in these patients is oxygen and efforts must be made to ensure that as much oxygen as possible is delivered to the patient's alveoli.

Pneumothorax

Definition

A pneumothorax is defined as the presence of air within the pleural cavity.

Physiological significance

The presence of a pneumothorax implies the existence of a communication between the pleural cavity and the tracheo-bronchial tree or, via a defect in the chest wall, between the pleural cavity and the atmosphere. Although this communication may not be evident at the time of diagnosis it represents a potential communication.

Air in the pleural cavity inevitably reduces the efficiency of ventilation. During spontaneous ventilation, mechanical effort is wasted as the result of air entering the pleural space rather than the lungs. During intermittent positive pressure ventilation a variable proportion of the tidal air maybe forced into the pleural cavity. Due to the lungs' elastic recoil inevitably the pleural space will be increased, causing a reduction in the volume occupied by the lung. Both these effects decrease the ventilation of that lung, thus creating some degree of ventilation/perfusion mismatch, or shunt. The degree of shunt is dependent on the amount of air in the pleural cavity, hence a large pneumothorax may give rise to hypoxaemia. A collapsed lung reduces the amount of normal lung which can be ventilated, and thus, if one is trying to ventilate the lungs with a fixed tidal volume, and the pneumothorax is not vented to the atmosphere, the inflation pressure will rise.

Pneumothoraces are often categorized as closed pneumothorax, open pneumothorax and tension pneumothorax (Fig. 2.6).

The danger associated with a communication between the lung or bronchus and the pleura is that further air will enter

PNEUMOTHORAX

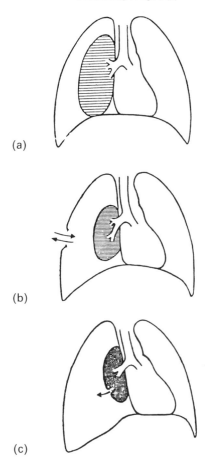

(a)

(b)

(c)

Fig. 2.6 The classification of pneumothoraces
    (a) Closed pneumothorax – intrapleural pressure negative
    (b) Open pneumothorax – intrapleural pressure atmospheric
    (c) Tension pneumothorax – intrapleural pressure positive

the pleural cavity. If air cannot return to the lung, i.e if a valve-like mechanism is operating, the pneumothorax will expand, causing it to compress the lung totally, and to increase the air pressure within the hemithorax. This is a tension pneumothorax. As the tension in the hemithorax increases it may push the mediastinum across the midline, impeding ventilation of the remaining lung and interfere with cardiac function. This can be rapidly lethal, and represents a medical emergency.

If there is a large enough hole between the pleura and the lung or bronchi, even if a drain is in situ in the pleura so that tension cannot be built up, it is possible for the leak from the hole to be so great that inflation of lung tissue becomes impossible.

An external or open pneumothorax is said to exist when it derives from an open defect in the chest wall caused by, for instance, a gunshot or stab wound. During the negative phase of spontaneous ventilation, air is sucked in via the wound, reducing the effectiveness of breathing – hence the classical description of a 'sucking chest wound'. If upper airway obstruction increases the negative intrathoracic pressures during attempted inspiration, the situation will become worse. The emergency management of open pneumothoraces is to prevent air passing through the wound. However, open pneumothoraces are only effectively relieved by positive pressure ventilation, provided the opening to the outside is patent.

Relevance to anaesthetists

Pneumothoraces are commonly created during surgery. This is inevitable in thoracotomies, and may occur accidentally during such procedures as nephrectomy, insertion of central venous lines and cervical sympathectomy.

The anaesthetist's use of intermittent positive pressure ventilation may encourage the development of a pneumothorax where none existed before. Patients with emphysematous bullae or pulmonary and chest trauma are particularly at risk in this respect, as are patients requiring high inflation pressures (e.g. in asthma and adult respiratory distress syndrome). However, any patient may at any time develop a pneumothorax, though it is rare for this to happen except in the above situations and where surgery close to the pleura is being conducted.

Intermittent positive pressure ventilation may convert a simple pneumothorax into a tension pneumothorax if an effective chest drain is not inserted. The anaesthetist may not be aware of the presence of the simple pneumothorax, and so a tension pneumothorax may seem to arise de novo. A qualitatively similar effect may be seen when nitrous oxide is used in the anaesthetic management of a patient with an undrained simple pneumothorax. This gas diffuses rapidly out of blood into the air-filled space, whereas nitrogen is only reabsorbed slowly. Thus the size of the pneumothorax increases, and when the lung is totally collapsed, pressure in the hemithorax will increase, giving rise to a similar clinical situation as a tension pneumothorax.

In general, closed pneumothoraces are made worse and more dangerous by intermittent positive pressure ventilation; however, it is usually the treatment of choice for open chest wounds.

Diagnosis and management

Pneumothorax looms large in the differential diagnosis of cyanosis, relative hypoxia and difficulty in ventilation during anaesthesia. The diagnosis is made by the clinical identification of air in the pleural cavity, reduced air entry into the lung and mediastinal shift. In trauma situations, subcutaneous emphysema is strongly supportive of the diagnosis. If time allows, diagnosis may be confirmed by chest radiography, although it can be difficult to detect quite large amounts of air in the pleural cavity unless the patient is erect or sitting up.

All tension pneumothoraces and all except the smallest simple pneumothoraces require drainage. In the case of a simple pneumothorax which is not compromising the patient's safety, there may be time for a formal insertion of a chest drain by an experienced person. The drain should be attached to a one-way valve, whether a 'flutter' valve, Heimlich valve, or more commonly, an underwater seal drain.

When a large simple pneumothorax causes significant hypoxaemia, or a tension pneumothorax has occurred, urgent drainage is required. The anaesthetist should insert a wide-bore intravenous cannula through the second intercostal space in the midclavicular line or through the fourth or fifth inter-costal space in the midaxillary line (Fig. 2.7). A rush of air will confirm the presence of a tension pneumothorax. A one-way valve should be connected to the cannula pending insertion of a formal chest drain.

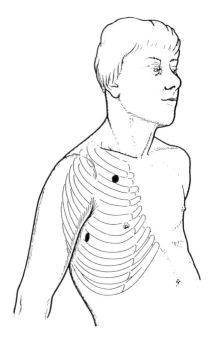

Fig. 2.7 Sites for the insertion of a chest drain:
        Second intercostal space, mid-clavicular line
        Fifth intercostal space, midaxillary line

When tension pneumothorax is a possiblilty, and a patient's clinical condition is rapidly deteriorating, the anaesthetist must not hold back in inserting a form of chest drain. Even if a tension pneumothorax is not present, the patient is unlikely to suffer significantly from the insertion of a 14 G intravenous catheter into the pleura. If a pneumothorax is present, this may be a life-saving procedure.

A particularly difficult clinical situation is where a large defect in the integrity of the tracheobronchial tree causes the major part of a patient's minute volume to be lost through the defect and out of a chest drain. Surgery is urgently required in this situation, and while surgical closure of the leak is being arranged and achieved, the anaesthetist must attempt to provide the patient with as much effective ventilation as possible. Though spontaneous ventilation is, in theory, more likely to be effective, it may be necessary to isolate the leak with the use of a double lumen endobronchial tube. This procedure, however, should only be undertaken by an experienced anaesthetist.

UNDERWATER DRAINS

The principles of underwater drains are simple and must be observed. The tube between the pleural cavity and the drain must be wide in order to minimize resistance and to allow air to be expelled easily from the pleural cavity. Its volumetric capacity must exceed one-half of the volume of the patient's maximum inspiration, or water from the bottle will be drawn into the chest. The height of water above the end of the underwater tube should not exceed 5 cm lest its resistance prevent air being blown off. The volume of water above the end of the underwater tube must be equivalent to at least one-half of the maximum inspiratory volume lest the seal be broken during a maximum inspiratory effort. The drain must always be at least 45 cm below the patient to avoid possible passage of fluid into the chest (Fig. 2.8) and the drainage tube must be clamped whenever the patient is to be moved. These conditions are best met by a wide-diameter, rather squat bottle. The disadvantage of this shape is that it renders accurate estimate of fluid drainage difficult, and therefore 1 litre graduated cylinders are often used. These are poorly designed for the purpose of underwater drains and must be changed if more than 200 dl of fluid has drained or if the level of fluid in the bottle is more than 5 cm above the end of the drainage tube. They are easily knocked over, breaking the seal, unless they are securely fastened.

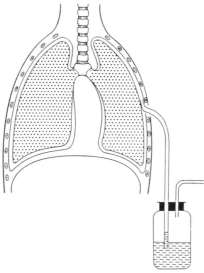

Fig. 2.8 An underwater seal chest drain in position

Cyanosis

Definition

Cyanosis is a blue coloration or either the skin or mucous membranes and is usually only evident when the concentration of reduced haemoglobin exceeds 5 g/dl. Although cyanosis may be caused by other mechanisms, e.g. methaemoglobinaemia, we shall consider only cyanosis caused by haemoglobin desaturation.

Physiological significance

The appearance of cyanosis during anaesthesia largely reflects venous desaturation. If a vascular bed (this can refer to part or all of the body) becomes cyanosed it therefore implies that one or more of the following changes is occurring:

1. The oxygen saturation of the blood supplying the vascular bed has been reduced, i.e. there has been a reduction in arterial saturation.
2. The blood flow through the bed has fallen, increasing the transit time of blood through the bed, and therefore the extent of oxygen extraction.
3. The oxygen demand of the tissues supplied by the vascular bed has increased, therefore increasing oxygen extraction.

As implied by the oxyhaemoglobin dissociation curve (Fig. 2.9), the proportion of haemoglobin which is desaturated is determined by the P_aO_2. In the normal individual, at a P_aO_2, of approximately 27 mmHg, 50 per cent of the haemoglobin will be desaturated. A patient with a haemoglobin of 14 g/dl will, at this P_aO_2, have 7 g/dl of desaturated haemoglobin and will be cyanosed. An anaemic patient whose haemoglobin is 8 g/dl will have only 4 g/dl desaturated, and may not appear cyan-

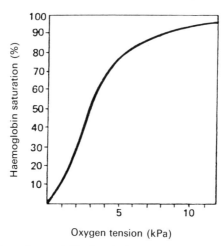

Fig. 2.9 The oxyhaemoglobin dissociation curve. The normal P50 is approximately 3.5 KPa, or 27 mmHg.

osed. Therefore, patients with a high haemoglobin will become cyanosed at a higher P_aO_2 than those with a low haemoglobin. The above does not imply that less note should be taken of cyanosis in a polycythaemic patient. Cyanosis in any patient indicates that tissue oxygenation may be inadequate. Conversely, an anaemic patient may not display cyanosis despite poor oxygenation.

Falling arterial saturation may be due to failure of ventilation or failure of perfusion.

Reduced oxygen saturation

Ventilation of the lungs with a hypoxic gas mixture, inadequate alveolar ventilation, and inappropriate distribution of inspired gases may cause a fall in saturation.

Decreased pulmonary blood flow may be due to right ventricular failure or outflow obstruction, reduced preload, right-to-

96

left shunt or pulmonary arterial obstruction. Ventilation/perfusion mismatch may be due to airways collapse, lung consolidation, the effects of gravity and anaesthesia.

Low blood flow.

A modest fall in cardiac output is common during anaesthesia. This is rarely sufficient to cause cyanosis as tissue demand is also reduced, and artificial ventilation reduces oxygen demand still further. Certain anaesthetic techniques, especially those which result in preload reduction, myocardial depression and high intrathoracic pressures, may significantly decrease cardiac output.

Straining and coughing during anaesthesia not only increase tissue oxygen demand as a result of exercise, but also cause a fall in cardiac output, venous congestion and reduced ventilatory gas exchange. As a result, tissue oxygen tension falls quickly and cyanosis appears.

If anaesthetic management cannot be held primarily responsible, pathological cardiovascular causes may be at the root of falls in cardiac output.

Peripheral vascular shutdown as a response to hypovolaemia, cold or pharmacological intervention may give rise to local cyanosis. However, at very low blood flows, skin and mucous membranes may appear pallid rather than blue.

The appearance of cyanosis can be mimicked by venous congestion as a result of positioning, increased intra-abdominal or intrathoracic pressure or physical venous obstruction.

Increased metabolic requirements.

Metabolic oxygen requirements usually fall during general anaesthesia, particularly if the muscles of respiration are paralysed. However, hyperthermia (and more rarely hyperthyroidism) causes an increase in oxygen demand during anaesthesia. In the postoperative period, shivering may cause dramatic increases in oxygen demand.

Diagnosis and treatment

The diagnosis of cyanosis is made by simple observation. If a pulse oximeter is being used, this should confirm that the cause is haemoglobin desaturation.

Ventilatory problems represent the commonest causes of cyanosis during anaesthetic management. These must be rapidly diagnosed or excluded. Hand ventilation with 100 per cent oxygen, bilateral chest auscultation to confirm air entry into both lungs and confirmation of the presence of an end-tidal carbon dioxide compatible with a tracheal gas sample should be the initial steps. If the lungs are being inflated effectively with 100 per cent oxygen, causes of V/Q mismatch or low pulmonary blood flow should be sought.

A significant fall in cardiac output as the cause of cyanosis should be accompanied by other associated stigmata, e.g. hypotension, a low pulse pressure and low end-tidal carbon dioxide. Steps should be taken to restore the cardiac output (see pp. 2–33). Peripheral vasoconstriction with low perfusion is associated with a large core peripheral temperature gradient, collapsed veins, etc. Local and peripheral cyanosis may not require active management, but if symptomatic of hypovolaemia or significant hypothermia, these should be corrected.

If cyanosis is thought to be due to a metabolic cause of increased oxygen demand, the core temperature should be monitored, and the possibility of the patient developing malignant hyperthermia should be kept in mind.

Postoperative shivering greatly increases oxygen demand, and may pose a further threat to the patient as cardiac output and hence the work of the heart may increase acutely. Preventive measures include avoidance of hypothermia and provision of adequate analgesia. Management of shivering includes the provision of added inspired oxygen and active warming.

Tachypnoea

Definition

The normal adult at rest has a respiratory rate of between 12 and 14 breaths/min. Tachypnoea may be defined as a persistent respiratory rate of more than 18 breaths/min.

Physiological significance

Within the context of anaesthetic management, tachypnoea can be considered to be a physiological response, usually to pain, to a derangement in blood gases or acid–base balance or a response to pharmacological intervention.

Minute volume is the product of respiratory rate and tidal volume. An increase in respiratory rate at a fixed tidal volume will therefore cause an increase in minute volume. This results in increased excretion of carbon dioxide, and a lowered P_aCO_2. This in turn will lead to a lower hydrogen ion concentration in the blood and hence a higher pH. Tachypnoea may therefore be used by the body as a response to hypercapnia or acidosis, tending to return P_aCO_2 and pH towards normal values. Tachypnoea is also a response to hypoxia, though in the normal patient this effect is only operative at low P_aO_2. If tachypnoea occurs in a patient with previously normal P_aCO_2 and pH, the resulting hypocapnia and alkalosis may have deleterious effects such as peripheral vasoconstriction and increased cerebrovascular resistance.

A painful stimulus given to an awake, lightly anaesthetized or inadequately analgesed patient will result in an increase in depth and rate of respiration.

Certain drugs sensitize the Hering–Breuer reflex, causing afferent suppression of inspiration, cutting it short and resulting in a more rapid respiratory cycle. Ether, trichloroethylene and halothane are particularly active in this respect if they are not balanced by central depression of the reflex by opiate drugs.

An increase in respiratory rate will increase energy expenditure and consequently oxygen demand will rise.

Aetiology

$P_a\text{CO}_2$ will rise if carbon dioxide production increases, excretion decreases or the inspired gas contains a significant proportion of carbon dioxide. A raised inspired carbon dioxide level may be due to contamination of the inspired gas with carbon dioxide or rebreathing of the patient's expired carbon dioxide due to the use of an inefficient breathing circuit or too low a fresh gas flow. Increases in metabolic activity due to hyperthermia, shivering or convulsions will increase carbon dioxide production and hence may give rise to tachypnoea. Reduced carbon dioxide excretion due to decreased tidal volume or increased respiratory dead space, whether anatomical, physiological or due to apparatus conformation, may also cause tachypnoea. Bicarbonate administration is a poorly recognized cause of tachypnoea; each 100 ml of 8.4 per cent sodium bicarbonate given produces 2.24 litres of carbon dioxide!

Hypoxia may give rise to tachypnoea. A review of the causes of hypoxia may be found on p. 95.

Tachypnoea may be a response to metabolic acidosis which has a variety of causes. Notable amongst these are lactic acidosis (often a result of tissue hypoxia, whether due to hypoxaemia or poor tissue perfusion, which includes the use of tourniquets), diabetic ketoacidosis, renal acidosis and loss of alkali from the gut.

Management

It is tempting to assume that tachypnoea occurring during anaesthesia is due to the combination of a painful stimulus and light anaesthesia or inadequate analgesia. Although this is the commonest cause, other causes of tachypnoea must be considered.

The onset of tachypnoea during anaesthesia may be related to the use of an inefficient breathing circuit, too low a fresh gas flow, the inadvertent administration of carbon dioxide, the administration of a particular volatile agent or an event such as the release of an arterial tourniquet. In these circumstances the cause is evident and treatment, if it is deemed necessary, can be directed to removing the cause. It is in those patients in whom the cause is less evident that the diagnosis must be established before it is simply assumed that the patient is too lightly anaesthetized and deeper anaesthesia is required.

A capnograph may establish whether the tachypnoea is an attempt to compensate for an increased P_aCO_2. If this reveals a high end-tidal carbon dioxide, ensure that the patient does not have an obstructed airway, that the breathing circuit does not have a large dead space, that the fresh gas flow is adequate and that the carbon dioxide is not being administered from the anaesthetic machine. The core body temperature may be measured to discover whether increased carbon dioxide production due to an acute rise in body temperature is the cause of tachypnoea. If present, this may herald the development of the rare condition of malignant hyperthermia.

If doubt still remains as to the cause of the tachypnoea, an arterial blood sample should be drawn for analysis to exclude metabolic acidosis.

If the tachypnoea persists in the absence of the above indications to a cause, and especially if other signs of inadequate anaesthesia are present, it is reasonable to administer a small dose of opiate or to deepen the anaesthesia.

Oxygen therapy in the recovery period

Physiological significance

There are times during the recovery from anaesthesia when it is desirable to increase the inspired oxygen content of air to compensate for hypoxia, or potential hypoxia, which may arise for a variety of reasons.

The alveolar oxygen content may be diluted by either nitrous oxide given off from solution in the body water (diffusion hypoxia) or a raised level of carbon dioxide due to hypoventilation. It may be a consequence of respiratory depression due to narcotic administration or inhalational anaesthesia, or muscular weakness due to residual paralysis with neuromuscular blocking agents. Hypoventilation is also a consequence of airway obstruction. Hypoxaemia due to ventilation/perfusion inequalities is common in the postoperative period, whether as an effect of the anaesthetic agents themselves, or as a result of small airways collapse and atelectasis. Greatly increased oxygen demand is associated with shivering in the recovery period, and oxygen therapy may be useful to prevent hypoxaemia in this situation.

However, oxygen therapy should not be used to compensate for the respiratory depression caused by drugs, except for short periods while steps are being taken to alleviate such respiratory depression. The treatment of significant respiratory depression associated with an inadequate minute volume is by artificial ventilation.

Disadvantages of oxygen therapy include a propensity to alveolar collapse due to high oxygen concentration and subsequent absorption collapse of alveoli, and the depression of hypoxic drive that may have significance for some patients with chronic pulmonary disease. High inspired oxygen concentrations for long periods may be associated with oxygen toxicity, it may mask hyperventilation and CO_2 retention. The application of an opaque mask may conceal the face and mouth, so that cyanosis or the presence of vomit may not be easily seen.

There is no doubt that postoperative oxygen therapy is given to many patients who do not require it and very often it is administered in an inefficient manner when it is of use. Unless an apparatus such as a Venturi mask is used (Fig 2.10(a)), where air entrainment with a low flow of oxygen can be controlled to maintain a given oxygen concentration even at high peak inspiratory flow rates, one cannot provide a predictable oxygen concentration in the inspired air. Most oxygen masks have a low dead space (Fig. 2.10 (b)(c)) (a high apparatus dead space in the presence of hypoventilation would further decrease effective alveolar ventilation, leading to a rise in P_aCO_2) and as a result, if the peak inspiratory flow rate exceeds a modest 15 l/min, the inspired oxygen is unlikely to be raised by more than 8–10 per cent. In practice, only if the mask is well sealed around the face, the oxygen flow is greater than 6 l/min, and the patient is breathing quietly, is an adequate effect obtained.

Most patients with severe postoperative hypoxaemia improve very little with routine oxygen therapy unless positive pressure oxygen is administered with a bag and mask, or after tracheal intubation. Increased respiratory dead space, shunt through unventilated alveoli, respiratory depression by narcotic drugs and residual muscle weakness are not effectively treated by placing an oxygen mask over the patient's face with a low flow of oxygen. That patients recover in spite of this treatment indicates the limited value of this therapy in these circumstances.

Management

Administration of oxygen therapy by low dead space, low flow masks in the recovery period is almost universal in anaesthetic practice. We would not encourage anaesthetists to stop this practice, but rather would stress the importance of careful consideration of the individual patient's likelihood of requirement for effective oxygen therapy and close observation in this period. If it is felt to be important to administer accurate concentrations of added oxygen, then apparatus designed to meet this criterion should be used. If hypoventilation is prolonged or of significant degree, then ventilation should be assisted or controlled.

The need for supplemental oxygen therapy often extends beyond the time taken for the patient to awake after an operation. Oxygen therapy extending some hours or even days beyond the end of anaesthesia should be considered, and if judged necessary, administered. Care should be taken to monitor the patient's respiratory status and the response of his or her oxygen saturation to the therapy.

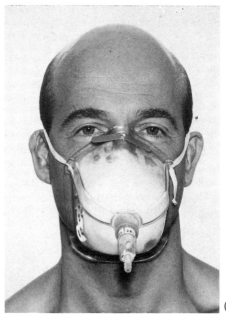

(a)

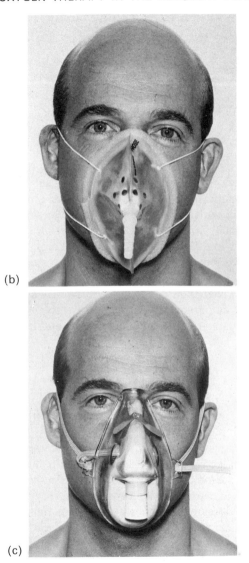

Fig. 2.10 Three commonly used oxygen masks
(a) Venturi mask (b) MC mask (c) Hudson mask

Hiccups

Definition

Hiccup is an involuntary and spontaneous eruption of short bursts of diaphragmatic spasm.

Physiological significance

Although hiccups may occur in uraemic states and in response to diaphragmatic irritation, their occurrence during anaesthesia is usually either a manifestation of a central stimulation of the medulla or a response to vagal, oesophageal or gastrointestinal traction. However, occasionally their occurrence is apparently without cause. Although hiccups cannot occur if the diaphragm is completely paralysed by a neuromuscular blocking agent, large doses of muscle relaxant are required to paralyse the diaphragm completely, therefore hiccups may occur despite apparently adequate surgical relaxation.

Management

Hiccups are very difficult to treat adequately in all circumstances. Hiccups due to drugs such as methohexitone are self-limiting and often associated with other signs of cerebral irritation such as coughing. In other circumstances the reflex can be obtunded by stopping the afferent stimulus (e.g. traction on the oesophagus), increasing the degree of central nervous system depression by deepening the anaesthesia or by giving large doses of narcotics, or by increasing the neuromuscular blockade still further. In certain circumstances the coordinated response of the central nervous system may be corrected by increasing afferent input. Nasopharyngeal suction, the brief administration of 5 per cent carbon dioxide or a small dose of droperidol have been described as being effective.

Violent hiccups can make intra-abdominal surgery difficult, and complaints from the surgeon can lead the anaesthetist to give a dose of muscle relaxant which may take a considerable time to wear off sufficiently to allow reversal. In practice, if the surgeon is persuaded to stop whilst the anaesthetic is deepened and a small top-up dose of muscle relaxant is administered, the hiccups usually disappear. Should the hiccups recur they are often so diminished as to be acceptable.

One-lung anaesthesia

We will not deal here with the placement of double lumen endobronchial tubes; other texts comprehensively cover this subject. We shall discuss problems encountered when establishing or conducting one-lung anaesthesia. Each subsection will consider a particular problem. Not all problems encountered during one-lung anaesthesia are directly related to the technique or the inflation of only one lung; the problems encountered in one-lung anaesthesia do not replace those encountered during endotracheal anaesthesia – they add to them.

PROBLEM: HIGH INFLATION PRESSURE DURING ONE-LUNG ANAESTHESIA

On transition from ventilating both lungs to ventilating just one lung, there is always an increase in inflation pressure. This is often in the region of 10–25 cm H_2O due to the shape of the pulmonary compliance curve. This can be reduced by decreasing the tidal volume and increasing the rate of ventilation, utilizing a more effective part of the compliance curve. However, the increase may be greater, and on occasions ventilation of the single lung may be impossible. The increase in inflation pressure usually occurs during the initial stages of one-lung anaesthesia. However, further rises may occur even when one-lung anaesthesia has been successfully established for some time.

Aetiology

Movement of endobronchial tube

Though the correct placement of the tube should be checked

by auscultation or fibreoptic bronchoscopy after the patient has been positioned on the table, it is still possible for it to move during surgery. Even small movements of the head can dislodge a previously well placed tube. A right-sided tube may have moved so that the right upper lobe is no longer being ventilated. The bronchial limb of the tube may have advanced so that the lumen is impacted against a bronchial wall.

Obstruction of endobronchial tube

It is surprisingly easy to kink double-lumen tubes, especially red rubber Robertshaw tubes which have been repeatedly autoclaved. Due to their relatively narrow lumens, obstruction with secretions or blood clots is not uncommon. Overinflation of the bronchial cuff may also cause tube obstruction.

Patient factors

The lung to be ventilated may be the seat of pre-existing disease reducing its compliance. Anatomical distortion of the carina may make accurate placement of the bronchial tube difficult without kinking. Secretions and blood clots distal to the tube can cause high inflation pressures. The transfer to one-lung anaesthesia can cause bronchospasm. Tension pneumothorax may be caused by high inflation pressure or attempts at central venous cannulation.

Management

If adequate inflation is impossible to achieve even when the tidal volume is reduced and the rate of ventilation increased, return to ventilation of both lungs. Auscultate the chest to exclude wheezing and ascertain whether all lobes of the lung are ventilating. Ventilation of the upper lobes is best confirmed by auscultating in the axillae, thereby minimizing transmitted breath sounds. However, even breath sounds in this area do not definitely confirm that the upper lobe is being ventilated. Let some air out of the bronchial cuff to exclude compression of the lumen by the cuff and herniation. Pass a suction catheter down both lumens of the tube to confirm patency and to allow removal of blood or secretions. Try withdrawing the tube a couple of centimetres and attempting inflation again.

If correct placement cannot be achieved by simple methods, it may be necessary to return the patient to the supine position and reintubate.

Certain patients, particularly those with chronic lung disease, will develop high inflation pressures on transfer to one-lung anaesthesia. For some it will not be practicable to continue one-lung anaesthesia for this reason. If lung resection in these patients is planned, it must be reconsidered. If surgery not involving lung resection is planned, for example oesophagectomy or thoracic aneurysm repair, the feasibility of performing the surgery without one-lung anaesthesia should be considered and discussed with the surgeon.

PROBLEM: HYPOXAEMIA DURING ONE-LUNG ANAESTHESIA

When initiating one-lung anaesthesia it is customary to increase the inspired oxygen (FIO_2) to 0.5 or greater. Despite this, hypoxaemia may occur. This may be made clinically obvious by the appearance of cyanosis, or may be detected with the use of pulse oximetry or blood gas measurements. The first indication of hypoxaemia may be the development of dysrhythmias or changes in blood pressure.

Aetiology

Provided that ventilation of the remaining lung is effective the most common cause of the hypoxaemia so often seen on starting one-lung anaesthesia is that perfusion continues to the non-ventilated lung, producing shunt (Fig. 2.11). The degree of shunt can be reduced by hypoxic pulmonary vasoconstriction (HPV) which develops. HPV is a response of pulmonary vessels to hypoxia which tends to reduce the blood flow to parts of the lung that are not well ventilated. Oxygenation also depends on the condition of the ventilated lung and the adequacy of its ventilation.

Management

If hypoxaemia occurs, increase the FIO_2, if necessary to 1.0. Beware, since the withdrawal of nitrous oxide that this involves may cause a lightening of anaesthesia. Adjust the concentration of inhalational agents or increase intravenous supplementation as necessary. Check that you are ventilating all lobes of the remaining ventilated lung. If the haemoglobin saturation is unacceptably low in spite of an FIO_2 of 1.0 (as is possible if there is a large shunt), the situation can only be helped by manoeuvres which:

1. Aim at oxygenating the blood passing through the non-ventilated lung and/or
2. Aim at decreasing the shunt through the non-ventilated lung by physical means.

Firstly, attach an oxygen source to a suction catheter and pass it into the lumen of the tube leading to the non-ventilated lung. Passing 5 to 10 l/min of oxygen through this may improve overall oxygenation. Beware of passing the catheter into the main bronchus during lobe resection or pneumonectomy as the catheter may become involved in the resection. Using too large a catheter may obstruct the escape of oxygen back through the lumen of the tube, causing the lung to become overinflated.

Further increasing the gas flow through the suction catheter will apply continuous positive air pressure CPAP (Figure 2.12)

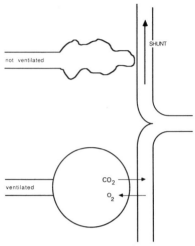

Fig. 2.11 Blood flow to non-ventilated lung is not oxygenated and constitutes true shunt

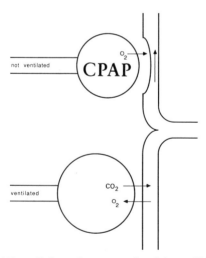

Fig. 2.12 CPAP applied to the non-ventilated lung. This may improve oxygenation by allowing gaseous exchange in the non-ventilated lung.

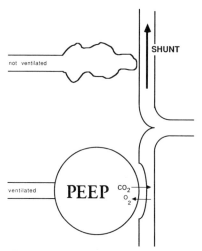

Fig. 2.13 PEEP applied to the ventilated lung. This may increase the shunt to the non-ventilated lung.

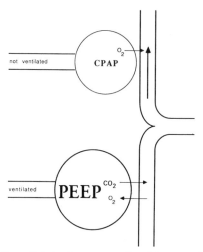

Fig. 2.14 CPAP applied to the non-ventilated lung, and PEEP to the ventilated lung.
This may further improve oxygenation but the balance of pressures has to be 'fine-tuned' to find an ideal match.

113

to the non-ventilated lung. Not only will this improve oxygenation of the blood passing through this lung, but it will also tend to decrease this shunt flow by a simple pressure effect. Consult with the surgeon before doing this as inflation of the lung may interfere with surgery. Other techniques of achieving CPAP to the non-ventilated lung are acceptable, but are not usually as easily available as the suction catheter technique.

Resist the temptation to apply positive end-expiratory pressure (PEEP) alone to the ventilated lung. This may cause a deterioration in oxygenation by increasing the shunted blood flow to the non-ventilated lung (Fig. 2.13). PEEP to the ventilated lung can, however, be effective if CPAP is simultaneously applied to the non-ventilated lung, thus resisting the blood flow redistribution (Fig. 2.14). Be mindful of the adverse effects of PEEP on venous return and hence cardiac output and blood pressure. The PEEP/CPAP approach can be 'fine-tuned' by adjusting airway pressures and finding out which combination best suits the need of the patient. If these manoeuvres are not effective, you should discuss with the surgeon whether it would be possible to perform the surgery without one-lung anaesthesia. Some specialized units may have the facility to initiate different ventilation modes, e.g. high-frequency jet ventilation to the upper lung combined with conventional-frequency ventilation with PEEP to the lower lung. However, we would not recommend this without the assistance of an anaesthetist with experience in such techniques and it is not always successful in correcting the hypoxaemia.

In the case of pneumonectomy, shunting to the unventilated lung is of course impossible after clamping and ligation of the pulmonary artery, and hypoxaemia can be largely avoided if this is performed early on in the procedure.

PROBLEM: CARDIOVASCULAR DISTURBANCE DURING ONE-LUNG ANAESTHESIA

Changes in blood pressure and dysrhythmias are common during one-lung anaesthesia. They may be a consequence of the physiological changes caused by one-lung anaesthesia; however, it is important to consider causes which are unrelated to one-lung anaesthesia.

Aetiology

Instigating one-lung anaesthesia and clamping of a pulmonary artery or its branches cause a significant increase in pulmonary vascular resistance. This in turn will cause an increase in right ventricular end-diastolic volume, and hence right atrial pressure. The hypoxic vasoconstriction in the collapsed lung results in the blood contained in that lung (200–500 ml) being transfused into the systemic circulation, increasing the venous pressure and subsequently the right atrial pressure. The resulting increase in right atrial volume may cause dysrhythmias due to stretching of the sinoatrial node area. For the first few beats, right ventricular output will be reduced, and therefore so will left ventricular output and blood pressure. In the patient with normal cardiac function and pulmonary vasculature, physiological responses will occur to normalize right heart output: a fall in pulmonary vascular resistance due to opening of parallel vessels in the lung and increased force of myocardial contraction resulting from increased myocardial fibre length (Starling's law). These will also tend to normalize right ventricular end-diastolic and right atrial pressures. Indeed at this stage it is not uncommon to observe a rise in blood pressure reflecting the increased systemic blood volume. Therefore, a transitory change in blood pressure accompanied by dysrhythmias is not surprising when initiating one-lung anaesthesia or at pulmonary arterial clamping. However a patient with limited right ventricular performance, ischaemic heart disease or pathologi-

115

cal changes associated with pulmonary hypertension, even though these were not clinically obvious preoperatively, may develop persisting hypotension and dysrhythmias associated with raised right atrial pressure indicative of right heart strain. Common dysrhythmias in this situation include tachycardia, multiple ectopic beats and atrial fibrillation.

Ventilation abnormalities will cause variations in P_aO_2 and P_aCO_2 which in turn can cause cardiovascular disturbances. Hypoxia may give rise to tachycardia and hypertension, followed by bradycardia, dysrhythmias and hypotension. Hypercapnia will cause tachycardia, hypertension and dysrhythmias. If, after a period of one-lung anaesthesia which involves significant shunting, there is a return to a smaller shunt due to resumption of two-lung ventilation, or resection of lung with pulmonary artery ligation, the previous relatively high minute ventilation will no longer be required to maintain carbon dioxide homeostasis; hyperventilation may therefore ensue.

Surgical contact with the heart, particularly common during left thoracotomies, can cause dysrhythmias, often in the form of atrial and ventricular ectopic beats. Accidental surgical compression of the heart or great vessels in the chest can cause decreased venous return and hence a reduced cardiac output.

Light anaesthesia will cause tachycardia and hypertension. This is more likely to occur during one-lung anaesthesia for two reasons. Firstly increasing the FIO_2 will decrease the percentage of nitrous oxide being used. Secondly, the increase in shunt will decrease the rate of uptake of inhalational agents.

Management

Most of the dysrhythmias and blood pressure fluctuations that occur during one-lung anaesthesia are short-lived and of little clinical importance. All life-threatening dysrhythmias or variations in blood pressure should be treated symptomatically. If the condition does not respond you can usually return to ventilation of both lungs.

Ensuring adequate oxygenation, ventilation and anaesthesia will eliminate the majority of cardiovascular disturbances. If surgical manipulation is the cause, ask the surgeon to take care to avoid pressure on the heart and great vessels. If these are excluded, and the patient's age or preoperative status suggest that right ventricular strain or failure is the root of the problem, careful consideration should be given to continuing procedures which include significant lung resection, as the patient may be condemned to permanent right heart failure postoperatively. If it is decided that the procedure should continue, and one-lung anaesthesia is absolutely necessary for the performance of the surgery – this is a rare combination! – steps should be taken to optimize right ventricular function. Inotropic agents will improve myocardial contractility, but at the possible expense of increased myocardial oxygen demand. Vasodilators will decrease pulmonary vascular resistance and right heart preload, at the possible expense of lower blood pressure. Digoxin or similar agents may be useful, particularly if fast atrial fibrillation presents a problem, but these drugs have slow onset times. Dysrhythmias can be treated along normal lines, but resist the temptation to use beta-adrenoceptor blockers to treat tachydysrhythmias or multiple ectopic beats in a situation where poor myocardial contractility may be at the root of the problem.

PROBLEM: THE NON-VENTILATED LUNG DOES NOT DEFLATE

Aetiology

There are two principal reasons for this: firstly, you may be unintentionally still ventilating the lung, and secondly, there is obstruction preventing gas from leaving the lung. Continued ventilation of the lung can be due to incorrect identification, connection or clamping of connectors to the two lumens of the endobronchial tube, incorrect tube placement, or inadequate bronchial cuff inflation. Obstruction to emptying of the lung, or of one of its lobes can be caused by kinking or blockage of the tube to that lung, by lung pathology, e.g. tumour or abscess obstructing a bronchus, or by secretions or blood achieving the same effect.

Management

Check all connectors and clamps and confirm that you are not ventilating the lung that you intend to deflate. Test the patency of the endobronchial tube to that lung; put a small amount of extra air in the bronchial cuff. Look at the lung; if it is not moving in time with the ventilator, it is likely that there is an obstruction to emptying. Pass a suction catheter down the lumen of the tube into the main bronchus and aspirate to remove secretions and blood. If these manoeuvres are not effective, it is likely that lung pathology is the cause.

SECTION THREE

Haematuria

Definition

The diagnosis of haematuria, i.e. the presence of red blood cells in the urine, requires microscopy, a technique which is rarely applicable to the anaesthetic context. During anaesthesia, haematuria is suspected if a red or brown discoloration of the urine leads the anaesthetist to believe that there are red cells or haemoglobin in the urine.

Diagnosis

Presuming that haematuria was not present preoperatively, the diagnosis of haematuria simply requires that other causes of red or brown discoloration of the urine should be excluded. These include:

Haemoglobinuria in patients with intravascular haemolysis
Urobilinogen in the jaundiced patient
Myoglobin in the patient with extensive muscle trauma (and occasionally following suxamethonium)
Porphobilinogen in patients with acute intermittent porphyria
Dyes derived from foodstuffs, e.g. beetroot
Drug causes, e.g. Dorbanex, rifampicin

If there is doubt, the diagnosis can be assisted by the use of proprietary urine analysis sticks which will give a positive reaction in the presence of haemoglobin.

Physiological significance

The presence of blood or haemoglobin in the tubules and

collecting ducts of the kidneys can, in itself, cause renal damage. The immediate significance of haematuria and hae-moglobinuria to the anaesthetist is the physical or pathophy-siological disturbance which can lead to this condition occur-ring during the course of an anaesthetic.

Aetiology

Haematuria or haemoglobinuria occurs during an anaesthetic for one or more of three reasons: trauma to the urinary tract, coagulopathy or haemolysis.

Trauma to the urinary tract

The act of urethral catheterization may cause haematuria and haematuria is a common consequence of many urological procedures.

The traumatized patient may have undiagnosed damage to the urinary tract which may not reveal itself until during an anaesthetic which is being administered for surgery to another part of the body. This is especially likely to occur after crush injuries to the abdomen and following road traffic accidents.

Non-urological lower abdominal surgery, particularly gynaecological or obstetric procedures, can cause haematuria.

Coagulopathy

If blood loss is extensive, and/or large volumes of stored blood are transfused, deficiency in clotting factors and platelets may cause haematuria in the absence of significant trauma to the urinary tract. This is usually associated with the observation of poor clotting in the surgical field. If the patient has a pre-existing subclinical coagulopathy, the blood loss and/or trans-fusion required to cause this will be less. If a patient has been receiving anticoagulant therapy preoperatively or if heparin has been given during the operation, haematuria may occur.

121

Haemolysis

The transfusion of incompatible blood or blood products may cause haemolysis. This causes haemoglobinuria unless it is so massive that tubular obstruction produces anuria.

Cardiopulmonary bypass is associated with a degree of haemolysis which is dependent on its duration. Haematuria is not uncommon following prolonged bypass procedures due to red cell damage.

The inadvertent transfusion of large volumes of hypotonic fluids, e.g. sterile water, causes haemolysis and haemoglobinuria. This may occur as a result of inspiration of large volumes of fresh water during drowning or from absorption of water if it has been used as an irrigant fluid during transurethral resection of the prostate (TURP) operations.

Patients with haemoglobinopathies may begin to haemolyse during an anaesthetic, e.g. if a sickle cell crisis is precipitated, or if oxidative drugs are given to a patient with glucose-6-phosphate dehydrogenase deficiency.

Investigation and management

There are many occasions when a mild to moderate degree of haematuria will come as no surprise to the anaesthetist, for instance during urological surgery, after a prolonged period of cardiopulmonary bypass, or after a traumatic catheterization. However, if the haematuria becomes apparent during surgery that involves or is in close proximity to the organs of the urinary tract, and if the haematuria is unexpected or of a greater degree than expected the anaesthetist should inform the surgeon, in case inadvertent damage has been caused or there is previously unsuspected trauma to the tract or kidney.

If haemoglobinuria is present and the patient is receiving a blood transfusion (especially if the haematuria is associated with acute cardiovascular changes such as tachycardia and hypotension) a transfusion reaction should be suspected, and the transfusion should be stopped. If this occurs during a period of extensive blood loss, sufficient to suggest a differential diagnosis of a coagulopathy combined with hypotension, a management decision will have to be made on the balance of probabilities. If there is doubt, the particular unit of blood being transfused at that time should be stopped, but active resuscitation should be continued, with crystalloid or colloid initially and with other units of blood once the compatibility of the blood provided for that patient has been checked.

Coagulopathy during extensive blood loss rarely becomes apparent until the patient has had a transfusion equal to at least one blood volume. It is suggested that it may occur more readily following surgery of the pancreas, lungs and prostate. If haematuria causes the anaesthetist to become suspicious that this is occurring, he or she should perform a platelet count and clotting studies on a sample of venous blood and provide platelet or clotting factor-rich blood fractions as indicated by the results of these studies. It may be deemed necessary to initiate transfusions before the results of these studies are available, but this is usually as a result of excess bleeding rather than haematuria.

If the haematuria cannot be explained readily, the anaesthetist should carefully review the patient's present condition and past medical history to ascertain whether there are other causes for haematuria, haemoglobinuria or discoloration of the urine, from other causes.

Oliguria and anuria

Definition

Oliguria is the failure to produce 400 ml of urine in a 24-h period. Anuria is the absence of urine production. These classical definitions need adaptation to the context of clinical anaesthesia. The adaptation is easy for anaesthetic anuria, this is the absence of urine production during the course of an anaesthetic. The definition of anaesthetic oliguria is distorted by the common notion that intraoperative urine output should be in the range of 0.5–1 ml/kg/h. For a 70 kg patient this extrapolates to a 24-h urine production of between 850 and 1700 ml, comfortably outside the classical definition of oliguria.

Diagnosis

Preoperative urinary catheterization is seldom performed for the express purpose of monitoring the urine output preoperatively. This is rightly so, as the risk to the patient of the insertion of a catheter must be justified by the potential benefits that will accrue as a result of the correct management of the physiological disturbances which give rise to the observed abnormality of rate of urine production.

Excluding purely surgical indications, urine output monitoring is therefore restricted to situations where the cardiovascular status of the patient is likely to change significantly, during prolonged operations where the vascular supply of the kidneys may be affected by the surgery, or in conditions associated with renal insufficiency, e.g. severe jaundice. Though there are exceptions to the above, the purpose of urine output monitoring should be considered to reflect either:

1. The cardiovascular status of the patient or
2. In the presence of a stable cardiovascular system, the functional status of the kidneys themselves.

With a catheter and drainage system in place, the diagnosis of anuria and oliguria should present no problem, providing an inadequate fluid load does not cause prerenal azotaemia, and the lower threshold of acceptable urine production has been decided.

Physiological significance

For adequate urine production the renal tubular mechanism must be functioning and an adequate head of pressure must be present to produce glomerular filtration. This requires viable renal tissue provided with an adequate oxygen supply to maintain enzymatic activity. It is possible to have viable kidneys with oliguria due to a low perfusing pressure, although if this is prolonged it may cause renal depression and oliguria even when the pressure is restored.

Aetiology

Artefactual oliguria and anuria due to blockage of the drain- age and collecting system for urine are common and must be distinguished from true anuria. If prolonged, the resulting back pressure may cause renal dysfunction. The kidney is primarily an organ of homeostasis and responds to demand. It will increase the volume output to dispose of excess intravascu- lar or extracellular fluid; conversely, it will reduce urine production if either of these fluid spaces is reduced.

Many patients present for anaesthesia in a dehydrated and sometimes hypovolaemic state due to the preoperative period of fasting or a facet of the disease process with which they present. Added to this are the metabolic effects subsequent to the stress of surgery, most of which cause a further degree of fluid conservation through the secretion of antidiuretic hor- mone, and hence reduced urine output. Anaesthesia itself tends to decrease renal blood flow. It is against this background of baseline fluid conservation by the kidneys that intraoperative urine output measurements must be viewed.

The anaesthetist must also be mindful of the patient's preoperative medical condition and renal function. A patient with renal impairment cannot usually be expected to excrete water and solutes as efficiently as one with normal renal function. A patient prone to congestive heart failure, deprived of the customary morning dose of diuretic therapy, may not readily pass water in spite of favourable cardiovascular conditions.

With the above comments in mind, the following should be considered as possible serious causes of a decrease in urine production during anaesthesia:

Prerenal causes

Dehydration
Hypovolaemia
Hypotension
Low cardiac output
Disruption to the vascular supply of the kidneys

Renal causes

After a period of renal ischaemia
In the jaundiced patient (hepatorenal dysfunction)
After administration of nephrotoxic drugs
Stress causing excessive antidiuretic hormone secretion
Myoglobinuria and haemoglobinuria

Postrenal cause

Obstruction to ureter or catheter

Investigation

Investigation of oliguria or anuria in the anaesthetic setting should always begin with confirmation that the collection and drainage system is functioning. If the abdomen is open, the surgeons can often confirm that the catheter is in the bladder, and that the bladder is empty.

The anaesthetist should then seek to confirm that the patient's cardiovascular status is such that the kidneys are likely to secrete urine. The blood pressure should be high enough to perfuse the kidneys adequately. A systolic pressure of above 90 mmHg should suffice for the healthy patient, but although urine production will be reduced below this level, it does not necessarily infer an impairment or renal tissue viability, merely an insufficient filtration pressure. However, those whose normal blood pressure is significantly raised may require a higher pressure. Poor cardiac output is also suggested by poor peripheral perfusion and a low pulse pressure. The diagnosis of hypovolaemia may be suggested by clinical obser-vation, the pulse and blood pressure, or by central venous or pulmonary capillary wedge pressures.

Careful reassessment of preoperative fluid intake and intraoperative blood loss may be useful in assessing the likelihood of hypovolaemia, as may consideration of the possibility of a significant third space loss.

Other factors, such as direct surgical effects on the vascular status of the kidneys, preoperative renal failure or dependence on diuretics, should be considered.

Management

The management of intraoperative oliguira or anuria should primarily be based on correction of the physiological derange-ments which are the root cause, should such be found.

The anaesthetist usually finds great solace in the observation and documentation that a patient is producing more than 0.5 ml/kg/h of urine during an anaesthetic, and certainly this observation indicates, in the majority of cases, renal function and viability. However, the reverse is not always true. The anaesthetist should, however, beware of two pitfalls:

1. That in pursuing this goal, the anaesthetist is 'treating the numbers' rather than looking to the physiological well-being of the patient as a whole, and that an adequate urine flow may be masking the kidney's inability to concentrate urine due to tubular derangements.
2. That overenthusiastic treatment of a causative factor such as hypovolaemia (by excessive fluid load or by mannitol) may confer a disadvantage to a patient prone to congestive cardiac failure, and therefore sensitive to volume overload.

The use of diuretic agents to create or increase urine production, other than those which act to increase renal blood flow such as mannitol, is seldom necessary, and it is the authors' opinion that such use should be restricted to situations where:

Hypovolaemia has been excluded (if necessary by invasive means, e.g. central venous pressure measurement).
Blood pressure is adequate.
Adequate time has been allowed since the achievement of the above to permit the appearance of urine.
Production of urine is deemed desirable to confirm renal viability, to increase urine flow following surgery to the ureter or renal pelvis, or to reduce cardiac filling pressures.

Convulsions

Convulsions during anaesthesia are very rare due to central sedation and muscle relaxation. However, they may occur during the recovery period when they may manifest as tonic uncoordinated limb movements or jerky twitching of the facial muscles and eyes. The diagnosis is difficult to make as full convulsive seizures are unlikely in patients who are often still sedated in the postoperative period. Convulsions must be distinguished from central stimulant effects of hypnotics like methohexitone and etomidate which can cause hiccuping, coughing and occasionally jerky limb movements which are self-limiting and usually only evident on induction; the non-convulsive athetoid movements caused by large doses of phenothiazines such as promethazine and perphenazine, and from the muscle rigidity associated with fentanyl and its cogeners. True convulsions may occur if toxic blood levels of local anaesthetic are achieved by inappropriate intravascular injection or overdose in an appropriate compartment.

An emergence phenomenon, commonly referred to as postoperative shivering, is seen after inhalational anaesthesia, particularly with halothane. It involves large muscles in uncontrollable movements which resemble shivering. It may be related to cold, and indeed, the patients often say they feel cold. There is some evidence that surface heating may reduce its severity. Postoperative shivering itself is not uncommon after operations during which the core body temperature has fallen. This is especially likely to occur if the procedure is of long duration, or if large volumes of cold fluid have been transfused. It differs from halothane shivering in causing finer muscle movements, erectopilae contraction and being self-limiting once the body temperature has been raised.

The ineffective attempts of a patient with residual muscle paralysis to open the eyes or move may also be mistaken for prodromal convulsive movements.

Physiological significance

The self-limiting halothane shivering, the muscle rigidity caused by fentanyl derivatives and the shivering due to cold have little primary significance for the central nervous system. Convulsive movements in the postoperative period are more significant as they may herald the development of true convulsions as the sedative effects of the anaesthetic wear off. If the patient has not previously been known to suffer from a convulsive disorder, the occurrence of convulsions may indicate a temporary or permanent disorder of brain function which may be associated with events during surgery, anaesthesia and recovery, or with the disease process for which the patient is being treated, or with problems related to it. Any centrally mediated convulsion greatly increases the oxygen demand of the brain, and may result in cerebral hypoxia and significantly raised intracranial pressure which may lead to permanent brain damage. The tonic contractions of skeletal muscles that occur during convulsions interfere with normal respiration and lead to inadequate ventilation.

Any greatly increased muscular activity, whether truly convulsive or due to shivering, increases oxygen demand. If it occurs in the immediate postoperative period it will do so at a time when the cardiac output is usually reduced well below normal and when lung ventilation/perfusion abnormalities frequently lead to some degree of arterial oxygen desaturation and metabolic acidosis. They are potentially dangerous as a result, especially in the elderly and those with cardiac disease or ischaemic organ disease.

Diagnosis and management

Any patient making uncoordinated movements in the recovery room should be observed carefully and consideration should be given to the cause of the movements. If the patient is making excessive muscle movements of any kind, whether true

130

shivering, halothane shivering, or minor convulsive movements, it is important to make sure that the increased oxygen demand is met and adequate ventilation is maintained. The inspired oxygen should be increased and assisted ventilation given if necessary. If the violence of the movements increases, a sedative with minimal respiratory depressive effects, such as a benzodiazepine, may be given. However, if this fails to correct the convulsive movements or if respiratory tidal exchange is inadequate, the patient should be paralysed and ventilated. In doing this, it may be wise to avoid agents which are associated with abnormal EEG activity, such as methohexitone and enflurane. Paralysis does not prevent seizure activity in the brain, and treatment with appropriate anticonvulsant agents should continue.

Concern has been expressed that a metabolite of atracurium, laudanosine, which has analeptic activity, may be responsible for convulsions. However, current evidence indicates that when atracurium is used in normal clinical doses, the laudanosine levels generated are well below those necessary to initiate convulsions.

Muscle rigidity

Occasionally a patient whose muscle tone appeared normal preoperatively may develop rigidity of some or all of his or her muscles during the course of an anaesthetic. This may be due to a primary muscle disease (e.g. dystrophia myotonica), diseases and drugs affecting the extrapyramidal system, or more rarely may be a harbinger of malignant hyperpyrexia. Muscle tone may also be increased by hypoxia, by increased secretion of catecholamines, by hypocalcaemia and by alkalosis.

Physiological significance

Muscle rigidity from whatever cause increases the metabolic demand enormously. When it involves a large proportion of the body muscles this can be equivalent to the energy usage during heavy exercise. Adequate ventilation and oxygenation should be assured while steps are taken to alleviate the rigidity.

Rigidity of the muscles of the head and neck may make maintenance of a clear airway or intubation very difficult. Rigidity of chest wall and abdominal muscles may make inflation of the patient's lungs impossible.

Aetiology and management

The drugs that produce idiosyncratic rigidity most commonly are fentanyl derivatives, especially alfentanil and sufentanil. The condition is usually self-limiting but if it continues, or if it occurs in a patient with cardiac disease, then it is necessary to paralyse the patient so that intubation and ventilation can be carried out. It may be prudent to administer a dose of hypnotic to ensure unconsciousness if this has not been produced by the narcotic. As alfentanil has been recommended as an induction agent for patients undergoing cardiac surgery, it is sensible to be prepared to treat muscle rigidity vigorously and early in these patients.

Suxamethonium may cause temporary rigidity in a region of the body, commonly the facial muscles. This disturbing condition is self-limiting but it may preclude early orotracheal intubation. It does not prevent ventilation provided the airway can be maintained. These patients will exhibit a similar reaction to a repeat dose of suxamethonium so that it is necessary to use a non-depolarizing muscle relaxant to achieve intubation. More widespread muscle rigidity with suxamethonium may be associated with myoglobinuria and can lead to renal tubular obstruction. Alkalinization of the urine is recommended, together with an infusion of mannitol to promote a diuresis from increased renal blood flow.

Some patients suffering from dystrophia myotonica demonstrate an increase in muscle tone in response to the administration of suxamethonium.

The phenothiazine drugs may produce a form of widespread muscle rigidity if an excessive dose is administered. This results from dopaminergic extrapyramidal depression caused by these drugs and is often associated with athetoid movements. The treatment is expectant – stop phenothiazine drugs, administer oxygen and ventilate if the condition is seriously impairing the ventilatory response to the increased oxygen demand.

Muscle rigidity is a very common (but not invariable) warning sign of impending malignant hyperpyrexia. It commonly follows halothane or suxamethonium, but many anaesthetic agents have been incriminated as being the triggering agent in this rare congenital muscle disorder. Should generalized muscle rigidity occur following induction of anaesthesia the patient's temperature and end tidal CO_2 should be monitored (in most patients with this condition the body warmth is obvious to anyone touching the patient). The blood pressure and ECG should be closely monitored. An intravenous infusion should be started and if the rigidity continues or the temperature rises active treatment should be started. The patient must be hyperventilated with oxygen and actively cooled; dantrolene sodium should be given intravenously and bicarbonate administered to reduce any acidosis that develops. Arterial blood should be monitored as biochemical derangements inevitably occur.

Inadequate muscle relaxation

Definition

There are times during anaesthetics for abdominal (and occasionally thoracic) operations when the surgeon comments on the inadequacy of the muscle relaxation. This may not be unexpected if it occurs towards the end of an operation when the anaesthetist is rightly reluctant to administer a top-up dose of neuromuscular blocking agent. However, it may occur when the anaesthetist believed relaxation to be adequate. In both circumstances it is necessary to assess the actual degree of neuromuscular block and to determine the best and most appropriate method of producing good surgical conditions.

Diagnosis

A gradual increase in the inflation pressure required to achieve the same tidal volume indicates a reduction in compliance often due to returning muscle tone in the chest wall and diaphragm. A gradual rise in end-tidal carbon dioxide may indicate decreased ventilation due to a decrease in compliance. The above subtle signs of the return of significant neuromuscular function are easily missed, and faced with a comment from the surgeon about the adequacy of muscle relaxation, the anaesthetist should be able to ascertain the degree of neuromuscular block by the use of a monitor of neuromuscular function such as a peripheral nerve stimulator. (Fig. 3.1)

If more than two twitches of the train-of-four are visible or palpable, this suggests the return of significant neuromuscular function. Vigorous post-tetanic potentiation confirms this.

It should be remembered that the diaphragm is relatively resistant to non-depolarizing muscle relaxants, and that diaphragmatic function may return before that of the facial muscles

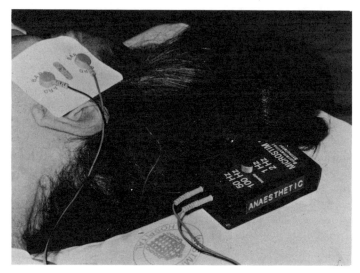

Fig. 3.1 (a) Simple peripheral nerve stimulator in position for stimulating facial nerve.

or adductor pollicis, especially if the patient has a normal or slightly raised $P\text{CO}_2$.

Management

It is pharmacokinetically unsound practice to give a long-acting non-depolarizing muscle relaxant shortly before the end of an operation as the blood level of the drug remains significantly raised for a period of time. This may cause difficulty in reversal of paralysis, and may give rise to residual curarization after the patient has been taken to the recovery room. Drugs rapidly cleared from the plasma, e.g. atracurium and vecuronium, can be given in a small dose to provide good relaxation for a limited period or a short surgical manoeuvre. If the degree of neuromuscular block is such that the first two twitches of the train-of-four have not returned, then deepening the anaesthetic with inhalational or intravenous agents may be sufficient to provide a quieter surgical field.

Anaesthetists may be tempted in this situation to administer a small dose of suxamethonium to provide intense muscle relaxation, for instance, for the closure of an abdomen. This temptation should generally be resisted. Firstly, a small dose is unlikely to suffice, as the presence of a non-depolarizing block increases the dosage requirements for depolarizing muscle relaxants. Indeed, a small dose of suxamethonium at this time may act like acetylcholine, causing a reversal of the existing block and reduction of muscle relaxation. Secondly, and most significantly, if an anticholinesterase is administered at a time when the suxamethonium is still active, its breakdown will be slowed, and its action greatly prolonged causing a dual block.

The value of a correctly applied neuromuscular block monitor during surgical procedures is considerable. It allows the anaesthetist to avoid overdosing the patient with relaxant and risking difficulty in reversal; it allows him to anticipate the return of muscle tone and it also allows him to know whether any difficulty experienced by the surgeon is really due to inadequate muscle relaxation. The earliest sign of returning neuromuscular conduction is elicited by a 50 Hz tetanic stimulus followed by a single twitch post-tetanic facilitation (PTF). If all four twitches of the train-of-four stimulation at 2 Hz are present and appear of equal strength, it is probable that complete reversal of neuromuscular block has occurred.

Hypothermia

Definition

Normal body temperature is maintained by homeostatic mechanisms which balance heat production by metabolic activities and heat loss. During anaesthesia and surgery many factors interfere with the normal homeothermic responses and a modest fall in skin and body temperature is quite usual. In the anaesthetized patient this does not necessarily constitute clinical hypothermia. However, if core temperature falls below 35°C then clinical hypothermia can be said to be present.

Aetiology

Anaesthesia deprives the body of its capacity to regulate body temperature which will tend towards the temperature of its surroundings. Operating theatres are almost invariably maintained at a temperature substantially below normal body temperature, therefore cooling is common during anaesthesia. This is exacerbated by such factors as heat and moisture loss if the patient is breathing cold dry gases, by the use of cold surgical preparation fluids; by the exposure of warm moist surfaces such as the peritoneum to the atmosphere, the infusion of cold intravenous fluids and by the cutaneous vasodilation that commonly accompanies anaesthesia. Rapid air changes in the operating room, especially laminar flow ventilation, can cause rapid and profound heat loss during anaesthesia. Muscle relaxation reduces the metabolic activity in, and hence heat production by, the muscles.

The rate and extent of cooling will depend on a variety of factors, notably the size and surface area-to-volume ratio of the patient, the temperature of the surroundings, the amount of the patient that is exposed to those surroundings, the length of the procedure and the use of techniques to prevent heat loss.

Physiological significance

Provided the fall in body temperature has been slow and the cooling even, a modest hypothermia to 35°C is without consequence in an adult.

As the body cools the heart beats more slowly, the cardiac output falls, peripheral vascular resistance increases, renal blood flow and urine secretion are reduced, metabolism in the liver is slowed and the minimum alveolar concentration (MAC) of volatile anaesthetic agents is reduced. Provided that the patient is adequately anaesthetized, oxygen consumption falls. The oxygen dissociation curve is shifted to the left and there is a decrease in end-tidal carbon dioxide due to a combination of decreased metabolic production and a fall in cardiac output. As a result, the minute volume requirements are reduced. Hypothermia can prolong the duration of effect of anaesthetic agents, and reduces the efficiency of coagulation mechanisms.

If the temperature falls to below 32°C or there is preferential cooling of the heart as a result of infused cold fluid reaching the heart, dysrhythmias may occur. Early ECG changes include the appearance of a J wave, sinus bradycardia, first-degree heart block and ST segment changes. Ventricular ectopic beats become increasingly common as the temperature is reduced; spontaneous ventricular fibrillation may occur at temperatures below 28°C.

Neonates and babies have a higher surface area-to-volume ratio than adults, and have poorly developed homeothermic mechanisms. For these reasons they are particularly prone to hypothermia during anaesthesia.

Patients suffering from hypothyroidism are prone to hypothermia.

Most fit adults will regain consciousness without ill effects at 35°C, but below this temperature consciousness may be obtunded.

Hypothermia during anaesthesia can give rise to shivering during recovery. Shivering greatly increases oxygen demand,

and causes a metabolic acidosis. When it occurs in the imme- diate postoperative period, it does so at a time when cardiac output, oxygen saturation and the oxygen-carrying capacity of the blood may be reduced. Once the patient has been re- warmed he should be observed for signs of possible hypovolae- mia which have been concealed by the vasoconstriction of the hypothermic state.

Management

Mild hypothermia may pose no threat to a fit patient. How- ever, when the patient is unfit, very young or elderly, or when the operation is likely to be long or involving substantial blood and fluid loss, it is a good idea to take steps to prevent hypothermia.

Keeping the operating theatre at a high temperature adds to the discomfort of the operating staff and is rarely justified except during neonatal anaesthesia. Heating blankets, heaters and humidifiers for inspired gases, blood warmers, warm irrigation fluids, wrapping up exposed parts of the patient etc. are all useful measures in preventing hypothermia.

The prevention of shivering during rewarming with the consequent risks of hypoxaemia and metabolic acidosis re- quires the patient to rewarm slowly. Active rewarming with radiant heaters may be useful. Vasodilation in a warm en- vironment will encourage rewarming, but the use of such drugs as alpha-adrenoceptor blockers, chlorpromazine or opiates has attendant risks which few anaesthetists would feel to be justified. The risks associated with shivering in the recovery period emphasize the importance of continued close observa- tion and monitoring even after the anaesthetic is completed.

If an elderly or unfit patient or one who has undergone extensive surgery is found to be significantly hypothermic at the end of an anaesthetic, consideration should be given to elective ventilation in an intensive care unit to allow careful monitoring and to ensure adequate ventilation and oxygenation until the patient is successfully rewarmed.

Hyperthermia

Definition

We shall define hyperthermia during anaesthesia as a patient core temperature greater than 39°C. The vasodilator effects of some anaesthetic agents may increase skin blood flow and give the impression of increased skin warmth when felt with the anaesthetist's hand. However, true hyperthermia can only be diagnosed with the use of a reliable calibrated thermometer, or similar device, measuring the temperature in such places as the nasopharynx, lower oesophagus, rectum or tympanic membrane.

Physiological significance

The rate of many metabolic processes catalysed by enzymes is proportional to temperature within a narrow physiological range. A small rise in body temperature will therefore cause a significant increase in the overall metabolic rate. This will cause a rise in oxygen demand, carbon dioxide production and the requirement for and usage of metabolic substrates. If the increased oxygen demand is to be met, oxygen flux must increase:

$$\text{Oxygen flux is proportional to cardiac output} \times Hb \times O_2 \text{ saturation}$$

Haemoglobin concentration cannot be increased in the short term and as oxygen saturation in the normal patient is above 95 per cent the increase in oxygen flux is achieved by an increase in cardiac output, which is accompanied by tachycardia and vasodilation. Patients who, due to age or heart disease, cannot easily increase their cardiac output may rapidly develop tissue hypoxia and acidaemia through the increase in anaerobic metabolism and lactic acid production. Those with a potential for ischaemic heart disease may develop myocardial ischaemia as a result of the increased myocardial oxygen demand produced by an increase in cardiac output.

In order to excrete the greater amount of carbon dioxide produced, alveolar ventilation will have to increase, and in the spontaneously breathing patient tachypnoea may be noticed. In the patient being ventilated at a fixed minute volume, or in those with pulmonary disease limiting their ability to increase alveolar ventilation, hypercapnia will result, leading to respiratory acidosis, dysrhythmias and further tachycardia and vasodilation. Patients who cannot increase oxygen uptake will become hypoxic.

Hyperthermia is associated with loss of intracellular potassium, and the hyperkalaemia which occurs may be aggravated by acidosis. Increased demand for substrate may cause hypoglycaemia if glucose stores cannot be adequately mobilized.

When body temperature exceeds 41°C cell damage occurs, as the structure and function of proteins and enzymes is dependent on the maintenance of temperature within a narrow physiological range. Brain damage is the usual cause of death attributable to hyperthermia alone.

Moderate hyperthermia may increase drug metabolism through its effect on enzyme activity.

Patients commonly experience a fall in core temperature during anaesthesia. If a modest increase in core temperature does occur, the fact that heat loss by conduction, convection and radiation is proportional to the temperature gradient with the environment usually prevents the development of physiologically significant hyperthermia.

An increase in core temperature may herald the development of malignant hyperthermia. This is an inherited disorder of skeletal muscle which can, after certain triggering circumstances, lead to greatly increased metabolism in the muscle, giving rise to excessive heat production, hypercapnia, hypoxia, hyperkalaemia and acidosis. The condition is triggered by a

number of agents, most noticeably halothane and suxamethonium. Malignant hyperthermia has a high mortality, and
although only a small minority of patients who show an
increase in core temperature will develop malignant hyperthermia, the diagnosis should be considered.

Aetiology

Hyperthermia may be associated with the following:

Drug effects, e.g. atropine in babies and infants, phenothia-
zines
Drug reactions
Bacteraemia or septicaemia
Blood transfusions (the effect of pyrogens)
Overenthusiastic attempts to prevent hypothermia
Faulty equipment used to prevent hypothermia, e.g. warm-
ing blankets, heater/humidifiers
Hyperthyroidism
Malignant hyperthermia

Management

The principles of management are to withdraw factors that
may be causing the hyperthermia, ensure adequate oxygenation and ventilation and encourage passive cooling while
monitoring the patient carefully.

Potentially causative drugs should be withdrawn, units of
blood being transfused should be stopped and retained for
laboratory investigation. If sepsis is suspected, blood cultures
should be taken and antibiotics considered. Devices for heating or prevention of cooling should be withdrawn. A pulse
oximeter and capnograph are useful monitoring devices, and if
acidosis is likely or suspected, arterial pH and blood gases
should be measured. The blood pressure and ECG should be
observed for evidence of cardiac decompensation. Appropri-

ate treatment of dysrhythmias, acidosis and hyperkalaemia should be initiated if these are demonstrated.

If, in spite of these measures, the core temperature continues to rise, active cooling may have to be employed. If malignant hyperthermia is suspected, triggering agents should be withdrawn, and if the diagnosis is supported by the demonstration of significant acidosis, dantrolene should be given.

Failure to recover consciousness

Definition

It would be normal to anticipate the return of consciousness within 10 minutes of the end of an operation. Failure to recover consciousness 60 minutes after the end of an anaesthetic requires investigation, unless an obvious preoperative or perioperative cause is apparent. In spite of apparent return of awareness, failure of memory and confusion may persist for some time postoperatively and do not necessarily require treatment.

Physiological significance

The speed with which recovery of the response to pain and to command occurs depends upon the preoperative status of the patient's central nervous system. It may also be affected by the surgery, intraoperative events and the pharmacokinetics of the drugs administered during anaesthesia. Full recovery of consciousness may vary according to the age of the patient (generally being longer in the elderly), and by pharmacokinetic effects of abnormal liver function, renal blood flow and protein binding. It is not unusual for some degree of mental impairment to be present for 24 hours after major surgery, manifesting itself as difficulty in concentration or temporary loss of recall of names. It is difficult to assess the contribution of the anaesthesia, surgery and postoperative medication to this phenomenon which is occasionally also found after major surgery under regional anaesthesia.

Physiology and pharmacology

Any condition reducing cerebral metabolism in the postoperative period is likely to cause delay in awakening from the anaesthesia. A fall in cerebral metabolism may be due to hypothermia, hypoxia or reduced metabolic substrates in the blood. Low cerebral perfusing pressure caused by systemic hypotension, an obstruction to venous outflow from the brain or from increased intracranial pressure will compromise cerebral function. Often a combination of factors is involved. Intraoperative cerebral hypoxia, due either to a fall in perfusion or to a critically lowered oxygen content of the blood, will affect postoperative recovery. If there has been an increased cerebrovascular resistance due to a low P_aCO_2 these effects will be exacerbated. Although in young non-anaesthetized subjects physiological autoregulation may compensate for decreased perfusion pressure or low oxygen content by causing a fall in cerebrovascular resistance, this mechanism is imperfect in the deeply anaesthetized and in elderly patients.

1. Drug-induced cerebral depression including a failure to lower the plasma concentration of anaesthetic agents to subhypnotic levels as a result of either overdose or pharmacokinetic factors is often a cause of modest delays in patients regaining full consciousness. This effect is often compounded by cerebral depression due to a raised P_aCO_2.

2. Pathological or pharmacological conditions that interfere with synaptic transmission and neurotransmitter release cause drowsiness and prolonged unconsciousness. Hypothermia below 32°C usually impairs consciousness.

3. High levels of plasma calcium or excessive use of calcium channel blockers may cause drowsiness by impairing neurotransmitter release, as may rapid falls in extracellular potassium.

4. A failure of glucose to reach the cellular enzymes will cause drowsiness and unconsciousness. This may be caused either by inadequate insulin in a diabetic or from very low blood glucose levels, usually associated with insulin administration not adequately covered with glucose.

5. Respiratory and metabolic acidosis either associated with carbon dioxide retention or with a low bicarbonate will disturb the function of the pH-sensitive intracellular enzymes and may cause unconsciousness.

6. Adrenocortical failure may present as hypotension and drowsiness or unconsciousness.

7. Physical damage either from direct trauma to the brain or from oedema resulting from past injury can cause unconsciousness. During surgery prolonged retraction of cerebral tissue may have the same effect.

8. The possibility of a cerebrovascular accident occurring during the operation should be considered as a cause of prolonged recovery of consciousness, especially if episodes of severe hypertension or hypotension complicated the surgical procedure.

9. Cerebral oedema from water intoxication is usually a slowly progressive condition but if associated with inappropriate antidiuretic hormone secretion, it may complicate recovery from anaesthesia.

Diagnosis

Hypotension and hypoxia occurring during an operation would alert one to this possible cause of cerebral damage – it is a practical aphorism that if the kidney continues to secrete urine, it is probable that the cerebral effects have been minimal. An alternative guide to prognosis is the ease with which regular normal respiration is restored. It is unusual for significant cerebral damage to occur without disturbing the pattern of normal respiration.

Raised intracranial pressure may be suspected if a possible cause was present preoperatively, such as a cerebral metastasis, or if the surgery may have interfered with cerebral venous drainage (such as tying the jugular veins when performing a bilateral block dissection of the neck). Confirmation of the diagnosis rests upon demonstrating papilloedema or a raised cerebrospinal fluid pressure; bradycardia, hypertension and periodic respiration should alert one to the possibility of raised intracranial pressure.

Cerebral oedema from water intoxication is suggested by a low plasma sodium level (below 110 mmol/l).

Intraoperative cerebrovascular accident is difficult to diagnose in the postoperative period as all the signs of an upper motor neurone lesion are usually present at the end of all operations. It should be suspected if no other cause of unconsciousness is found and if there has been an episode of extreme hypertension during the operation.

Hypoglycaemia, metabolic acidosis, calcium and potassium aberrations can be diagnosed by plasma analysis. Hypercarbia, either as a result of inadequate alveolar ventilation or the administration of high concentrations of carbon dioxide, should be suspected if there is tachypnoea, tracheal tug, a bounding pulse and peripheral vasodilation.

The commonest causes of a slow return of consciousness postoperatively are drug overdose or pharmacokinetic failure to lower plasma drug concentration often complicated by carbon dioxide retention. The administration of a dose of narcotic shortly before the end of the operation should alert one to this as a cause of slow return of consciousness. In the presence of poor renal blood flow, narcotic metabolites may cause respiratory depression. A slow respiratory rate suggests this diagnosis, which can be confirmed by the response to an injection of naloxone. Tracheal tug is commonly a sign of central nervous system depression associated with respiratory or metabolic acidosis. If volatile anaesthetics have been administered in a concentration greater than two mimumum alveolar concentrations they may well cause slow arousal. Obese patients have an enormous capacity to absorb these drugs and take many hours to reach true equilibrium – they may also take a long time to lower their plasma levels sufficiently to allow full return of consciousness.

Management

The first principle of management is to try to obtain conditions in the patient that are as close to physiological normality as possible. Fluid and electrolyte imbalance should be corrected, carbon dioxide, oxygen and glucose levels should be normal and the blood pressure should be maintained at a mean of 70–90 mmHg. Once this is achieved specific treatments can be applied, although, as in many situations in medicine, provided viable physiological conditions are maintained, recovery is just as likely to occur without drug intervention or specific remedies. Whilst naloxone is useful to reverse opiate depression, analeptics and other drugs seldom alter the ultimate course of recovery. However, if a focal cerebral lesion, such as an intracranial tumour or localized haemorrhage, has been diagnosed, modest hyperventilation may be necessary.

Failure to breathe after reversing neuromuscular blocking agents

Definition

This presents at the end of an operation in one of two ways:

1. In spite of the administration of an adequate dose of anticholinesterase, there is no respiratory effort.
2. Following reversal by anticholinesterase, respiratory effort is seen but the tidal volume is inadequate.

Physiology and pharmacology

The automaticity of the respiratory centre is affected by afferent impulses from the carotid body; by the pH of the cerebrospinal fluid and $P_a\text{CO}_2$ of the perfusing blood, and by higher centres. All of these afferent mechanisms as well as the respiratory centre itself may be affected by anaesthesia and its physiological consequences. The efferent pathway via the phrenic nerve to the diaphragm may be blocked at the neuromuscular junction. Normal respiration necessitates a functioning respiratory centre, normal pH and $P_a\text{CO}_2$ and an intact efferent pathway.

Mechanical impairment of ventilation due to obstruction of the air passages or diaphragm, or from pneumo- or haemothorax must first be excluded as causes of respiratory inadequacy or reduced tidal exchange.

Failure to make any respiratory effort is usually due to central depression of the respiratory centre by drugs or hypocarbia. Prolonged (over 5 min) complete failure to make respiratory effort is seldom due to reflex influences upon the centre, although temporary inhibition can be caused by afferent suppression, i.e. irritation of the larynx or trachea. In patients with severe airways disease and with significant preoperative hypoxic drive, a normal or raised $P_a O_2$ may depress reflex respiratory drive, making the re-establishment of normal respiratory effort difficult to achieve postoperatively.

The causes of hypoventilation include those affecting the respiratory centre such as drugs, hypocarbia, an anoxic insult to the respiratory centre, acidosis, loss of hypoxic drive due to high $P_a O_2$ and to failure to complete the reversal of the neuromuscular block.

Physiological significance

In the absence of adequate gas exchange due to inadequate tidal volume, artificial ventilation must be maintained. A 50 per cent nitrous oxide:oxygen mixture should be used to maintain unconsciousness. Artificial ventilation should be continued whilst an effort is made to correct any metabolic or respiratory abnormality and whilst any residual drug effect has time to be dissipated. It is often preferable to accept the necessity for intermittent positive pressure ventilation for 12 hours or more rather than to resort to compounding any pharmacological problem by the use of antidotes and analeptics.

The return of sufficient respiratory effort to achieve an adequate tidal volume is not in itself sufficient evidence of the patient's safety as it may be associated with insufficient muscle power to protect the airway by coughing and swallowing. The ability of a patient to raise his or her head off the pillow for 30 s and to sustain a cough is considered to be evidence of adequate return of neuromuscular function. If a peripheral nerve stimulator is available, the restoration of the fourth-to-the-first ratio of the train-of-four to above 70 per cent is convincing confirmatory evidence.

Diagnosis and treatment

It is first necessary to demonstrate that the cause of failure to restart normal respiration is not due to a cause other than residual neuromuscular block.

To determine whether it is due to inadequate P_aCO_2 to stimulate the respiratory centre, 7 per cent carbon dioxide should be administered for 2 min or rebreathing allowed to occur until the end-tidal carbon dioxide settles at 7 per cent. Ideally this should be confirmed by arterial blood gas carbon dioxide partial pressures.

To determine whether there is depression of the respiratory centre's response to carbon dioxide by opiate drugs, naloxone should be administered. Remember that naloxone is a short-acting agent and opiate respiratory depression may return after its offset.

If the patient had preoperative pulmonary disease, the possibility of reduced hypoxic drive causing respiratory depression can be tested by cautiously reducing the inspired oxygen content to 21 per cent. Adequate oxygenation during this manoeuvre should be confirmed by pulse oximetry or arterial blood gas analysis.

To demonstrate the state of neuromuscular conduction, stimulate a peripheral nerve such as the ulnar nerve in the forearm or the facial nerve in front of the tragus of the ear using a peripheral nerve stimulator (Fig. 5.1). The response to four supramaximal stimuli at 2 Hz should reveal the presence of all four twitches and these should be of equal force. It is very difficult to quantitate this response without a recording device of some kind, but the four-to-one twitch response should exceed 70 per cent. The response to 20–50 Hz tetanic stimulation will be a well maintained contraction if neuromuscular conduction is normal. Any fade or post-tetanic enhancement suggests residual block (Fig. 5.2). If the patient is conscious, the ability to squeeze two fingers of the anaesthetist's hand or to raise the head off the pillow for 30 s suggests that the block is reversed.

If there is any evidence of residual block it is reasonable to administer a further 2.5 mg of neostigmine (with atropine),

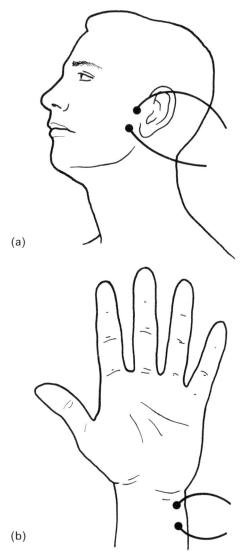

(a)

(b)

Fig. 5.1 (a) Position of stimulating electrodes over facial nerve
(b) Position of stimulating electrodes over ulnar nerve

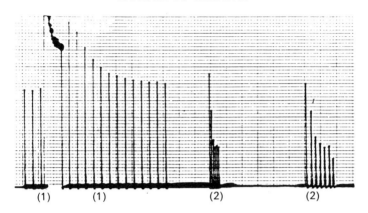

Fig. 5.2 Post tetanic faciliation (1) and train of four (2) in a partially curarised patient.

provided that it is certain that the residual paralysis is not associated with the use of suxamethonium in the presence of low cholinesterase activity.

If this fails to reverse the neuromuscular block as demonstrated by the train-of-four response, the patient should be ventilated whilst an effort is made to reduce the plasma level of neuromuscular blocking agent. As most neuromuscular blocking agents are excreted to a greater or lesser extent in the urine, it is often helpful to know if urine is being produced. Bladder catheterization will indicate whether it is likely to be profitable to increase renal blood flow and excretion by the infusion of 10 per cent mannitol and fluid. Reversal of persistent neuromuscular block often becomes possible once good urine flow is established.

The possibility that aminoglycoside antibiotics may have contributed to the neuromuscular block will be evident from the perioperative history. This condition can sometimes be partly alleviated by the use of 10 ml of 10 per cent calcium gluconate i.v. The agent of choice in this condition and in overdose of calcium channel blockers is 4 amino-pyridine;

however, due to its low therapeutic ratio, it should only be used with great caution.

If the patient is suspected of having a dual block following the use of large amounts of suxamethonium or in a patient with deficient cholinesterase activity – this may cause a short-lived partial reversal when 10 mg edrophonium is administered – the patient should be electively ventilated for about 2 h to allow the drug to be excreted. Mannitol is often helpful in promoting excretion of the drug via the kidneys.

Residual neuromuscular blockade should never jeopardize a patient's life if adequate ventilatory support is maintained; however, injudicious use of drugs to reverse the condition may cause complications and compromise ultimate recovery.

Postoperative restlessness

Physiological significance

Postoperative restlessness always deserves careful consideration. It may be due to one or more of a variety of causes.
Common causes include increased afferent input to the brain
from the pain of surgery, or from other discomforts such as a
full bladder, a tight wound dressing or an infusion that has
tissued. This, combined with cerebral depression due to the
drugs used during anaesthesia, may prevent a rational or
useful response by the patient, resulting in agitation and
restlessness. It may also be due to cerebral confusion due to
drugs, cerebral hypoxia or to lack of orientation due to
unfamiliar surroundings, e.g. eyes being bandaged or ears
covered. Agitation in the postoperative period may be a result
of inability to co-ordinate movements properly due to the
residual effects of neuromuscular blocking agents.

Diagnosis and management

Before making the easy and most likely diagnosis that the
cause of the restlessness is the pain of surgery and necessitates
administration of an opiate drug, it is essential to be quite
certain that there is no element of hypoxia, airway obstruction
or hypovolaemia. To give an opiate to a patient who is hypoxic
or hypovolaemic postoperatively may reduce the restlessness
but it will dangerously increase the hypoxia and may worsen
hypotension. There is little doubt that the administration of
opiates to patients with postoperative hypoxia or hypovolaemia, especially if due to haemorrhage, in the belief that their
restlessness was due to pain has caused patient deaths. A pulse
oximeter is useful in making the diagnosis of hypoxia but
unfortunately oxygen saturations less than 98 per cent are
common in the postoperative period and do not necessarily

indicate respiratory depression. In the presence of pain, ventilation is often increased and vasoconstriction may occur, making pulse oximeter readings difficult to interpret. However, should the oxygen saturation fall below 90 per cent following an opiate, the patient should be carefully monitored and given added inspired oxygen. It may become necessary to administer naloxone to reverse the action of the opiate drug. This is often associated with a return of pain.

Usually the diagnosis of postoperative hypoxia will be made on clinical grounds – laboured, obstructed breathing, tracheal tug, poor respiratory excursion and low tidal volume and a failure to breathe deeply on command. The colour of the patient may indicate hypoxia but as most postoperative patients, and especially those who are restless, will be receiving oxygen supplementation, hypoventilation and respiratory obstruction may not produce significant desaturation. The pulse, blood pressure, skin perfusion and temperature may indicate hypovolaemia which is often associated with concealed blood loss in the postoperative phase.

Restlessness due to drugs, especially if combined with a disorientating experience, such as waking up with eyes bandaged or nasal passages obstructed, may occur, especially in the elderly. In these patients further depressant drugs merely delay their recovery. The treatment should be symptomatic to prevent patients from hurting themselves whilst an explanation of their condition is repeated in an effort to orientate them. Postoperative confusion due to drug withdrawal or in an alcoholic does not usually manifest itself until 12 h after the procedure.

Restlessness due to incomplete reversal of neuromuscular blockade can be detected using a nerve stimulator. Clinically restlessness is associated with jerky uncoordinated movements, the use of the frontalis muscles to open the eyes and the inability to raise the head off the pillow for 30 s. This cause of postoperative restlessness should be managed along the lines given on pp. 154–158.

POSTOPERATIVE RESTLESSNESS

When all other causes of restlessness have been eliminated it is reasonable to conclude that the agitation is due to pain. Before an opiate is administered it should be determined that the pain is from the operative site and is not a warning sign of some imminent surgical complication such as bleeding into a tissue space, too tight a bandage or swelling of a limb encased in plaster. The patient's bladder should be percussed and felt to make sure that a full bladder is not the reason for agitation. Only when one is confident that pain due to the operative wound is the cause of the patient's restlessness should a postoperative analgesic be administered.

If an opiate analgesic is chosen, the dose administered should be adequate to control the patient's pain but not to cause undue respiratory depression in the unstable postoperative period. The dose may be difficult to predict and therefore the common practice of prescribing postoperative medication before the operation is to be deprecated. If there is doubt as to the dose of analgesic it is reasonable to administer it in divided doses intravenously, waiting 3–5 min between doses to observe the effectiveness of the analgesia and the degree of respiratory depression produced.

Inadvertent intra-arterial injection

Physiological significance

Many intravenously administered drugs are irritant and if injected into an artery can cause a reaction both in the artery and in the small vessels in the distribution area of the artery. Unless the reaction is such that severe arterial spasm ensues, the active agent will eventually pass into the venous system and will cause its systemic effect. However, there is likely to be a delay in onset of action due to the slow rise of central compartment concentration of the drug, a reduced peak plasma concentration and a less effective response.

The local action of the drug on the arterial wall may cause damage to the intima, leading to thrombosis at a later date. The reaction in the tissues supplied by the artery may be in the nature of a histamine-evoked triple response with oedema and erythema, or if the spasm is intense it may cause gangrene or tissue necrosis.

Drugs may be irritant due to the pH at which they are solubilized, e.g. thiopentone (especially if the concentration is greater than 2.5 per cent) or due to an irritant solubilizing agent such as intralipid (e.g. Diazemuls). Mannitol 10 and 20 per cent solutions are irritant by virtue of their hyperosmolarity.

Diagnosis and treatment

The delay in onset of action of thiopentone may be the first indication that the injection is intra-arterial. Blanching or blushing of the area supplied by the artery may draw attention to the accident. This is more likely to occur if the injection has inadvertently been given into an aberrant artery on the back of the hand or a branch of the ulnar artery. The treatment depends to some extent on the agent used but it is always sensible to dilute the offending agent by flushing the artery with normal saline. If the operation can be abandoned or the reaction is severe, heparinization may be considered to prevent clotting and reduce the risk of later thrombosis. It should be continued for 3 days.

The use of alpha-blockers such as tolazoline may be useful if the needle is still in the artery, as may be the injection of papaverine and procaine. If the arterial spasm is marked a sympathetic block should be performed; in the case of intra-arterial injection in the arm, this will be a stellate ganglion block. Elevation of the hand to reduce oedema and analgesia to cover what is invariably a painful episode may be required.

Inadvertent subcutaneous injection

Physiological significance

There can be few, if any, anaesthetists who have not given an accidental subcutaneous injection of an anaesthetic agent. Usually only very small amounts of air and drug are given before it is noticed. Such injections may have no more significance than discomfort for the patient if he is awake. However, the consequences of subcutaneous injection will have greater implications if the volume is large, the solution is irritant, or if the agent injected will constitute a significant depot of drug that will be slowly absorbed into the system circulation.

A large volume of fluid injected subcutaneously may cause discomfort, and if, due to the site of injection, it cannot spread, may cause tissue ischaemia through a pressure effect and subsequent skin and subcutaneous tissue necrosis. Subcutaneous injection of large volumes of crystalloid into an area where the above does not easily occur, e.g. the axilla, has been used in the past as a therapeutic manoeuvre for rehydration where venous access is impractical or impossible.

Highly irritant drugs such as thiopentone and fluids such as mannitol may cause local pain and inflammation, but where the volume is large or the concentration high, severe local vasospasm may result, leading to blanching, skin ischaemia and necrosis, which in severe cases may lead to extensive skin loss and the need for skin grafting.

Subcutaneous injection of a drug will establish a depot of the drug which will be slowly absorbed into the systemic circulation. The rate at which this is absorbed will be affected by the mass of drug injected, the blood flow to that area of the skin, and how the drug itself affects local skin blood flow. In general, when compared with intravenous or intramuscular injection of the same amount of drug, the time of onset of its effect will be longer, the peak plasma concentration will be lower, and the duration of action of the drug will be longer. This may be of particular relevance for potent drugs that are administered in small volumes, e.g. muscle relaxants and opiates.

Aetiology

The aetiology of accidental subcutaneous injection is the misplacement of a needle or cannula, usually one that is intended to be intravenous. If this occurs in an area where the veins are superficial and the skin cover is thin, e.g. the dorsum of the hand, subcutaneous injection is likely to be recognized early, providing that the site of injection is carefully observed during injection. Injections into areas where veins are deeper and skin cover is thicker should be conducted with particular care, confirming correct positioning by aspiration and close observation of the injection site.

Management

If accidental subcutaneous injection occurs or is suspected, the injection should be immediately stopped. If the volume is small, the drug is not irritant, or the depot effect of the drug is unlikely to be clinically significant, it may not be necessary to take any action other than removing the needle or cannula and establishing correct intravenous access.

If the drug is irritant and the volume injected is significant, its concentration can be reduced by injecting non-irritant isotonic fluid through the needle or cannula. Be careful to inject a fluid in which the drug is soluble in order to avoid precipitation of the drug concerned. One potential hazard of this technique is that the drug may spread, extending the area of the effects of the irritant drug. Infection is always a risk in these patients due to the distension of tissue space and the likelihood of necrotic tissue. As a result it is wise to consider giving antibiotic cover.

If the depot effect is thought to present a potential risk to the patient, hyaluronidase may be injected subcutaneously. This enzyme will encourage breakdown of connective tissue locally, and will enhance the spread of the drug, increasing its rate of absorption into the systemic circulation. Increasing limb blood flow by warming the limb or performing a sympathetic block will aid drug uptake. The potential prolonged effect of the drug should be appreciated, and appropriate monitoring and management instituted.

If the volume of fluid injected subcutaneously is a cause of concern, hyaluronidase may have some effect, though it is likely to be small due to its dilution. If practical, the limb should be elevated to encourage passage into the venous and lymphatic drainage systems. Surgical advice may have to be sought, and pressure-relieving procedures such as fasciotomy may be considered.

The site of any subcutaneous injection should be closely observed, not only intraoperatively, but also postoperatively so that if any adverse local effects occur appropriate management can be conducted early.

Vomiting and aspiration

The aspiration of stomach contents into the lung during induction, preoperatively or immediately postoperatively is a common cause of avoidable 'anaesthetic' death. This may follow active vomiting in the presence of a depressed laryngeal protective mechanism, or in circumstances that overwhelm the normal defence mechanism. Passive regurgitation and aspiration is probably common in anaesthetic practice, but in only a minority of instances does it cause clinical effects.

Physiological significance

In order to vomit, the patient must first inspire and then close the glottis. The lungs are thus filled with air which builds up intrathoracic pressure so as to maintain the diaphragm low in the abdomen. This acts as a roof against which the muscles of the abdomen contract to establish an intra-abdominal pressure which exceeds that in the thorax. This straightens the angle between the stomach and the oesophagus, which normally functions as a sphincter, and allows forced evacuation of stomach contents into the pharynx. In the normal patient the glottis remains closed throughout this process and vomit is expelled from the mouth.

The stimulus to vomiting may come from the higher centres (visual, auditory, etc.), from the vestibular apparatus, and from a chemoreceptor trigger zone. Often in anaesthesia it is the result of gastric distension and irritation or pharyngeal stimulation. Vagal stimulation (e.g. eye and external auditory meatus) may also cause nausea and vomiting.

Vomiting is often preceded by such warning signs as swallowing and builds up to a full inspiration followed by closure of the glottis. It is commonly accompanied by signs of vagal activity: pallor, sweating and bradycardia.

It is quite possible that minor degrees of tracheal soiling

occur during vomiting and are usually without significance; this is especially likely in debilitated and elderly patients where the laryngeal reflex is depressed.

It is the inhalation of acid or irritant material, the inhalation of particulate matter of sufficient size to block minor bronchi or the sheer volume of the aspirant that makes the condition serious. Blockage of the bronchi by particulate matter will cause immediate V/Q disturbances and if not removed will lead to pneumonitis, bronchopneumonia and lung abscess. Large volumes, even if they are clear fluids, can cause reflex bronchospasm, fluid absorption disturbances and problems associated with proteins, fats and other contained substances. The acid aspiration syndrome, as its name suggests, is caused by aspiration of acid. It results in a chemical pneumonitis with many of the hallmarks of adult respiratory distress syndrome and carries a high mortality.

It follows that for vomiting to occur there must be material in the stomach or in the distended small bowel, that the patient must be able to breathe in and close the glottis, he or she must have good abdominal muscle power and the glottic protective reflex must be obtunded.

Stomach contents

It is not possible to empty the stomach completely with any certainty. A large-bore stomach tube (size 10 oesophageal) can be used and will usually remove most of the fluid and smaller food matter. However, once removed, as is often recommended before anaesthesia, the stomach may fill retrogradely from the small bowel when the intra-abdominal pressure rises. Starvation alone does not empty the stomach; indeed, resting gastric juice is on average 150 ml and highly acid.

Even producing vomiting by use of an emetic such as apomorphine does not guarantee that the stomach will not refill from the distended small bowel. What is surprising is not

168

that aspiration of vomit occurs but that it does not occur more frequently.

Inspiration and closure of glottis

A once popular technique of dealing with patients at risk from aspiration of vomit was to make them rebreathe or to administer carbon dioxide before induction of anaesthesia. The respiratory drive was then too active to allow patients to hold their breath. As a result, they could not vomit. However, if any reflux of stomach contents occurred their laryngeal protection was absent. This technique is not recommended!

Obtunding glottic reflex

Depression with narcotics and hypnotics, local anaesthesia and small (even priming) doses of muscle relaxants are all more potent than volatile anaesthetics at obtunding this reflex. However, induction with a volatile anaesthetic is more likely to provoke vomiting.

Methods of minimizing risks of aspiration

Reducing stomach contents. No solid or semisolid food should be taken within 6 h of a planned operation. Fear, morphine, pain, pregnancy etc. delay gastric emptying, as may diseases such as pyloric stenosis or bowel obstruction. Children should be starved for their normal interval between meals or snacks. Minimal clear fluids, i.e. 20 ml/h are permissible if the patient is uncomfortably dry. Stomach contents can be reduced in volume by aspiration through a wide-bore stomach tube. The tube should be removed before anaesthesia is induced. Metoclopramide may increase the rate of gastric emptying and increase lower oesophageal sphincter tone.

Reducing acidity of stomach contents. Antacids such as magnesium trisilicate and sodium citrate may be given 30–60 min before the operation or sodium bicarbonate just before induction. H_2-blockers such as cimetidine given intravenously 2 h preoperatively increase the pH of gastric fluid and reduce the volume.

If there is a risk of aspiration of vomit, a technique of induction that obviates the need to inflate the patient, i.e. preoxygenation, should be used. It is virtually impossible to avoid inflating the stomach when using a bag and mask to inflate the lungs.

Cricoid pressure (Sellick's manoeuvre). Correctly applied compression of the oesophagus between the cricoid cartilage and the vertebrae will obstruct the oesophagus. The pressure must be firm. Do not apply pressure during active vomiting as oesophageal rupture is possible due to the pressure generated below the cricoid ring. The backwards pressure on the cricoid can bruise the larynx and often makes visualization of the cords difficult. It is doubtful if the pressure used by most anaesthetists during this manoeuvre is really adequate – cases where it has been carried out and the endotracheal tube has entered easily into the oesophagus demonstrate how difficult it is to obstruct this structure.

Use of head-down or lateral position. This used to be the treatment recommended, and still has much to commend it. It is difficult to aspirate vomit against gravity. A 15° head-down tilt does not make intubation difficult whereas the lateral position does. If used properly it is very safe; the worst complication is that vomit will soil the nasopharynx and spill over the anaesthetist! It has been said that this position increases the risk of regurgitation following administration of a muscle relaxant. It is probable that most cases of so-called regurgitation following suxamethonium are the result of active vomiting occurring due to too hasty attempts to intubate before the relaxant had actually taken effect. Passive regurgitation may lead to aspiration if the vomit is forced into the tracheobronchial tree by the use of mask intermittent positive pressure ventilation.

Awake intubation. This method of dealing with a potential risk of aspiration is widely practised in the USA. It necessitates some local anaesthesia of the upper airway and sedation of the patient. It is relatively easy in enfeebled and elderly patients but requires considerable patience, skill and co-operation to succeed in young strong adults. Too much local anaesthesia may obtund the protective reflex and too much sedation makes aspiration possible.

None of the above techniques is foolproof unless carried out with great care and attention to detail. It is essential always to preoxygenate patients at risk in order to have maximum time to carry out these manoeuvres unhurriedly. Inflation of the stomach with anaesthetic gases must be avoided. Adequate doses of hypnotics must be administered, unless using awake intubation, and time must be allowed for muscle relaxants to work effectively before intubation is attempted. A good working suction apparatus must be available and an assistant should be present during the induction and intubation.

Management

If a patient vomits, he should immediately be placed head-down, and preferably in the left lateral position. This encourages drainage of the vomit away from the larynx.

Oxygenation and ventilation must take priority over all other treatment. As positive pressure ventilation with a mask carries the risk of encouraging soiling of the airway, it is recommended that the patient should be intubated. This will allow ventilation and aspiration of vomit from the trachea and bronchi and will protect the lungs from further vomiting. In certain circumstances, such as when a patient with a full stomach vomits after extubation and is demonstrating an ability to protect the airway effectively, an experienced anaesthetist may elect not to intubate the patient. However, intubation with a cuffed tracheal tube is the only sure way to protect the airway from aspiration of stomach contents in the anaesthetic setting.

If there is doubt as to whether tracheal aspirate contains stomach contents, it can be tested with litmus paper, which will turn red when in contact with acid.

When significant aspiration of vomit has occurred, the patient should be transferred to an intensive care unit so that he or she can be monitored and, if it becomes necessary, ventilated. Even if the extent of aspiration is thought to be minimal, the patient should be observed closely and reassessed regularly, as the signs and symptoms of acid aspiration syndrome may take some hours to develop. A chest X-ray may be useful in assessing the extent of lung soiling and to this end it is helpful to have a comparison with a preoperative X-ray or, failing this, one taken as soon after the incident as possible.

If the patient's condition permits, bronchial toilet may be performed using saline or dilute bicarbonate solution. The lavage should be carried out until clean fluid is returned. The administration of large doses of steroids has been recommended and may be tried. Antibiotic cover should be instituted to prevent secondary infection.

Drug reactions

Definition

In the clinical setting, it is difficult to differentiate a true abnormal response to the administration of a drug from side-effects, overdose effects or a drug interaction. To the anaesthetist who is presented with a patient who is responding in an unexpected way to an anaesthetic agent, it is the physiological effects of that response and the implications it has for the continuing management of that patient that are important.

We shall define a drug reaction as an unexpected response occurring in a patient which may be attributable to an abnormal reaction to an anaesthetic agent.

Physiological significance

Local reactions to drug injection are common. Pain and blanching often occur with the injection of induction agents, especially if they are injected into small veins on the dorsum of the hand in anxious vasoconstricted patients. This is found particularly with methohexitone, propofol and etomidate. Erythema or urticaria at the site of the injection or tracking along the veins of the arm may imply the release of histamine or other vasoactive substances. This is common with such agents as pethidine, atracurium and tubocurarine.

Erythematous rashes, particularly noticeable on the neck and upper trunk (blush area), occur, as may widespread flushing over most of the body. The former is not uncommonly seen with suxamethonium, and the latter with tubocurarine. These may be associated with patches of urticaria.

These responses may have little or no physiological impact. However, they should alert the anaesthetist to the fact that a more significant response may be occurring. The large-scale release of histamine and other vasoactive and bronchoconstrictive substances is involved with more serious reactions, described as anaphylactic or anaphylactoid. The hallmarks of these reactions are hypotension, bronchospasm, urticaria and, occasionally, glottic oedema. These four are not always present together; a drug reaction can consist of only one. The hypotension and bronchospasm can vary in severity from mild to immediately life-threatening.

Drug reactions also include dysrhythmias, abnormal movements and muscular rigidity. As these are covered elsewhere we will not deal specifically with them in this section.

Management

Pain and blanching distal to the injection site on injection should immediately alert the anaesthetist to the possibility of inadvertent intra-arterial injection (pp. 162–164). If these reactions or localized erythema or urticaria occur with a drug with which they are not normally associated, or occur in a patient with multiple allergies or an atopic disposition, it would be wise to suspend administration of the drug if this can be done safely, and choose a drug with a similar action from a different pharmacological group. More widespread cutaneous reactions are more likely to be associated with severe drug reactions.

The anaesthetist should, as ever, monitor the patient's blood pressure after induction, and if hypotension occurs, should immediately establish intravenous access and give a plasma expander, whether crystalloid or colloid. Colloid is often recommended for the hypotension of allergic drug reactions, as the fall in blood pressure is in part due to plasma loss from the circulation. If bronchospasm occurs, the patient should be intubated and ventilated with 100 per cent oxygen. Halothane or another inhalational agent may be used as it is an effective bronchodilator which will keep the patient anaesthetized.

Management of the bronchospasm and hypotension should follow the guidelines given elsewhere in this book. Rarely, the drug reaction may be so severe as to necessitate the administration of adrenalin. Steroids may be given, as may antihistamines, but they are unlikely to be effective immediately.

It is often difficult to identify which particular drug was responsible for an anaphylactoid or anaphylactic reaction, as anaesthetic drugs are often given in rapid sequence. Patients can be tested for sensitivity to anaesthetic agents, and results may prove of great importance for the patient's future anaesthetic management. It is sensible therefore to test all patients in whom an anaphylactic response has occurred so that the provoking agent can be avoided in future.

It is difficult to tell whether an unexpected response is a truly abnormal one. The anaesthetist should observe and monitor every patient closely, responding appropriately to any physiological disturbances that occur. If you feel strongly that the patient did have an abnormal response to a particular agent, a record of this should be made in the notes. Unfortunately many patients become labelled as allergic to a particular drug when what has occurred may not have been drug-induced or may have been a result of overdose or sensitivity to a particular agent. If it is suspected that this is the case a very small test dose of drug may be given alone and the effects closely monitored. It should never otherwise be assumed that a warning about a patient's previous allergic response is incorrect.

Index

INDEX

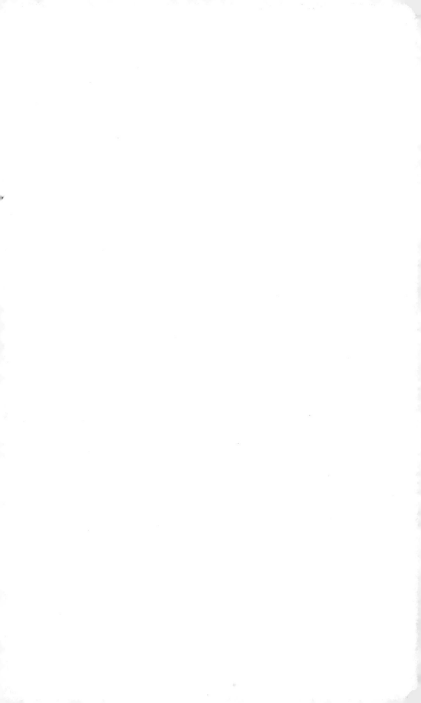